LEGALIZATION OF MARIJUANA NEEDS YOUR HELP.

National Organization for the Reformation of Marijuana Laws.

OFFICIALLY NOTED

Free the weed!

*Marihuana,
the Forbidden
Medicine*

Marihuana, the Forbidden Medicine

LESTER GRINSPOON, M.D.

AND JAMES B. BAKALAR

Yale
University
Press
New Haven
and
London

Published with assistance from the Kingsley Trust Association Publication Fund established by the Scroll and Key Society of Yale College.

Designed by Nancy Ovedovitz and set in Berkeley Old Style type by Tseng Information Systems, Inc. Printed in the United States of America by Vail-Ballou Press, Binghamton, N.Y.

Library of Congress Cataloging-in-Publication Data
Grinspoon, Lester, 1928–
Marihuana, the forbidden medicine / Lester Grinspoon and James B. Bakalar.
  p. cm.
  Includes bibliographical references and index.
  ISBN 0-300-05435-1
  1. Marihuana—Therapeutic use. I. Bakalar, James B., 1943–
II. Title.
RM666.C266G75 1993
615'.323962—dc20   92-34882
                         CIP

A catalogue record for this book is available from the British Library.

The paper in this book meets the guidelines for permanence and durability of the Committee on Production Guidelines for Book Longevity of the Council on Library Resources.

10   9   8   7   6   5   4   3

To the courageous contributors
who share their stories in this book

The rejection of any source of evidence
is always treason to that ultimate rationalism
which urges forward science and philosophy alike.

—Alfred North Whitehead

Contents

Preface   ix

1   The History of Cannabis   1

2   Cannabis as a Medicine   24

     Cancer Chemotherapy   24

     Glaucoma   40

     Epilepsy   58

     Multiple Sclerosis   67

     Paraplegia and Quadriplegia   81

     AIDS   85

     Chronic Pain   92

     Migraine   106

     Pruritis   109

     Menstrual Cramps and Labor Pain   113

     Depression and Other Mood Disorders   115

     Other Medical Uses   126

     In Defense of Anecdotal Evidence   133

3   Weighing the Risks   137

4   The Once and Future Medicine   155

     Index   177

Preface

When I began to study marihuana in 1967, I had no doubt that it was a very harmful drug that was unfortunately being used by more and more foolish young people who would not listen to or could not understand the warnings about its dangers. My purpose was to define scientifically the nature and degree of those dangers. In the next three years, as I reviewed the scientific, medical, and lay literature, my views began to change. I came to understand that I, like so many other people in this country, had been brainwashed. My beliefs about the dangers of marihuana had little empirical foundation. By the time I completed the research that formed the basis for a book, I had become convinced that cannabis was considerably less harmful than tobacco and alcohol, the most commonly used legal drugs. The book was published in 1971; its title, *Marihuana Reconsidered*, reflected my change in view.

At that time I naively believed that once people understood that marihuana was much less harmful than drugs that were already legal, they would come to favor legalization. In 1971 I confidently predicted that cannabis would be legalized for adults within the decade. I had not yet learned that there is something very special about illicit drugs. If they don't always make the drug user behave irrationally, they certainly cause many non-users to behave that way. Instead of making marihuana legally available to adults, we have continued to criminalize many millions of Americans. About 300,000 mostly young people are arrested on marihuana charges each year, and the political climate has now deteriorated so severely that it has become difficult to discuss marihuana openly and freely. It could almost be said that there is a climate of psychopharmacological McCarthyism.

One indication of this climate is the rise in mandatory drug testing, which is analogous to the loyalty oaths of the McCarthy era. Hardly anyone believed that forced loyalty oaths would enhance national security, but people who refused to take such oaths risked loss of their jobs and reputations. Today we are witnessing the imposition of a chemical loyalty oath. Mandatory, often random testing of urine samples for the presence of illicit drugs is increasingly demanded as a condition of employment. People who test positive may be fired or, if they wish to keep their jobs, may be involuntarily assigned to drug counseling or "employee assistance" programs.

All this is of little use in preventing or treating drug abuse. In the case of cannabis, urine testing can easily be defeated by chemical alteration of the urine or substitution of someone else's urine. Even if the urine sample has not been altered, the available tests are far from perfect. The cheaper ones are seriously inaccurate, and even the more expensive and accurate ones are fallible because of laboratory error and passive exposure to marihuana smoke. But even an infallible test would be of little use in preventing or treating drug abuse. Marihuana metabolites (breakdown products) remain in the urine for days after a single exposure and for weeks after a long-term user stops. Their presence bears no established relationship to drug effects on the brain. It tells little about when the drug was used, how much was used, or what effects it had or has. Like loyalty oaths imposed on government employees, urine testing for marihuana is useless for its ostensible purpose. It is little more than shotgun harassment designed to impose outward conformity.

Another aspect of psychopharmacological McCarthyism is suggested by the response to a publication in the May 1990 issue of *American Psychologist.* Two psychologists at the University of California, Berkeley, reported the results of a rigorous longitudinal study of 101 eighteen-year-olds whom they had been following since the age of five to examine the relation between psychological characteristics and drug use. The results showed that adolescents who had engaged in some drug experimentation (mainly with marihuana) were the best adjusted. The authors comment:

> Adolescents who used drugs frequently were maladjusted, showing a distinct personality syndrome marked by interpersonal alienation, poor impulse control, and manifest emotional distress. Adolescents who had never experimented with any drug were relatively anxious, emotionally constricted, and lacking in social skills. Psychological differences between frequent drug users, experimenters, and abstainers could be traced to the earliest years of childhood and related to the quality of their parenting. The findings indicate that (a) problem drug use is a symptom, not a cause, of personal and social maladjustment, and (b) the meaning of drug use can be understood only in the context of an individual's personality structure and developmental history.[1]

This study suggests that the current anti-drug campaign ("Just Say No") is misguided because it concentrates on symptoms rather than underlying problems.

A hue and cry began immediately. The director of a San Francisco drug prevention program said that it was irresponsible for researchers to report that "dabbling with drugs was 'not necessarily catastrophic' for some youths and may simply be a part of normal adolescent experimentation." A physician who directs the adolescent recovery center of a metropolitan hospital asked, "What does this do to the kids who made a commitment to be abstinent? Now they're being told they're a bunch of dorks and geeks. You can imagine how much more peer pressure is going to be put on them." An author writing in *Pride Quarterly* (Summer 1990) stated: "Based on the experiences

---

1. J. Shedler and J. Block, "Adolescent Drug Use and Psychological Health: A Longitudinal Inquiry," *American Psychologist* 45 (May 1990): 612–630.

of only 101 subjects, all living in San Francisco, the study still drew national attention due to its outrageous conclusion." "Unfortunately," continued the writer, "the permissive thinking which surfaced in the California study will continue to exist in the United States until truly effective drug education reaches beyond the elementary classroom. However, too few educators themselves have seen the latest discoveries about the health consequences of drug use."[2] It was all reminiscent of Stalinist party-line criticism of science.

In spite of the illegality of marihuana and the prejudices against it, large numbers of Americans continue to use cannabis regularly. Once considered a youthful indulgence or expression of youthful rebellion, marihuana smoking is now a common adult practice. Millions have smoked marihuana for years, and many of them will continue to smoke it for the rest of their lives. They are convinced that they are harming no one else and not harming themselves, if at all, as much as cigarette smokers or alcohol drinkers are.

Most users, in fact, believe that marihuana enhances their lives— a subject rarely discussed in print. In more than two decades of research, I have read a great deal about the potential harmfulness of cannabis (much of it nonsense) and very little about its value. Although this value has several aspects, medical use is one of the most important and one that has been seriously neglected. I have come to conclude that if any other drug had revealed similar therapeutic promise combined with a similar record of safety, professionals and the public would have shown far more interest in it. The largely undeserved reputation of cannabis as a harmful recreational drug and the resulting legal restrictions have made medical use and research difficult. As a result, the medical community has become ignorant about cannabis and has been both an agent and a victim in the spread of misinformation and frightening myths.

What follows is largely a book of stories, because most of the evidence on marihuana's medical properties is anecdotal. Some day the

2. J. Diaz, "Furor over Report of Teenage Drug Use," *San Francisco Chronicle,* May 15, 1990; *Pride Quarterly* (Atlanta), Summer 1990, pp. 1, 8.

systematic neglect of the research community will be remedied and the authors of a book on the medical uses of marihuana will be able to review a large clinical literature. James Bakalar and I hope to reverse prejudices, relieve ignorance, and help prepare the way for that research by exploring the known and potential therapeutic uses of this remarkable substance.

This is a book by two authors and many contributors. Most of the contributors were recruited by word of mouth or by referral, but some came to our attention through testimony they gave before Drug Enforcement Agency Administrative Law Judge Francis Young during the 1986 hearings on the rescheduling of marihuana. Robert Randall and Alice O'Leary of the Alliance for Cannabis Therapeutics helped us locate some of these patients. We are indebted to Kevin Zeese of the Drug Policy Foundation for, among other things, providing us with a transcript of the hearings. Our manuscript benefited immensely from critical readings by Kenneth Arndt, M.D., Ann Druyan, John Gehring, M.D., David and Betsy Grinspoon, Norman Jaffe, M.D., Simeon Locke, M.D., Susan Milmoe, Carl Sagan, Richard Schultes, and Arnold S. Trebach. Our project was also aided in diverse ways by Peggy S. Alcorn, Beth Banov, Del Cogswell Brebner, Elizabeth Case, Leslie Druyan, Paul Geissler, James Johnson, Jeff Moore, June Riedlinger, Alexander Shulgin, Lewis L. Van Hoosear, M.D., and Lennice Werth. We are especially indebted to Heather L. Erskine, who so competently assisted us at every stage of development of the manuscript and whose lovely demeanor was never compromised by seemingly unending revisions.

Lester Grinspoon, M.D.

1 History of Cannabis

The marihuana, cannabis, or hemp plant is one of the oldest
psychoactive plants known to humanity. It is botanically classified as a member of the family Cannabaceae and the genus *Cannabis*. Most botanists agree that there are three species: *Cannabis
sativa*, the most widespread of the three, is tall, gangly, and
loosely branched, growing as high as twenty feet; *Cannabis indica*
is shorter, about three or four feet in height, pyramidal in shape
and densely branched; *Cannabis ruderalis* is about two feet high
with few or no branches. There are also differences among these
species in the leaves, stems, and resin. According to an alternative classification, the genus has only one highly variable species,
Cannabis sativa, with two subspecies, *sativa* and *indica*. The first
is more northerly and produces more fiber and oil; the second is
more southerly and produces more of the intoxicating resin.

Cannabis has become one of the most widespread and diversi-
fied of plants. It grows as weed and cultivated plant all over the
world in a variety of climates and soils. The fiber has been used
for cloth and paper for centuries and was the most important
source of rope until the development of synthetic fibers. The
seeds (or, strictly speaking, akenes—small hard fruits) have been
used as bird feed and sometimes as human food. The oil contained in the seeds was once used for lighting and soap and is now
sometimes employed in the manufacture of varnish, linoleum,
and artists' paints.

The chemical compounds responsible for the intoxicating and medicinal effects are found mainly in a sticky golden resin exuded from the flowers on the female plants. The function of the resin is thought to be protection from heat and preservation of moisture during reproduction. The plants highest in resin therefore grow in hot regions like Mexico, the Middle East, and India. When the reproductive process is over and the fruits are fully ripe, no more resin is secreted.

The cannabis preparations used in India often serve as a folk standard of potency. The three varieties are known as *bhang, ganja,* and *charas.* The least potent and cheapest preparation, bhang, is produced from the dried and crushed leaves, seeds, and stems. Ganja, prepared from the flowering tops of cultivated female plants, is two or three times as strong as bhang; the difference is somewhat akin to the difference between beer and fine Scotch. Charas is the pure resin, also known as hashish in the Middle East. Any of these preparations can be smoked, eaten, or mixed in drinks. The marihuana used in the United States is equivalent to bhang or, increasingly in recent years, to ganja.

The marihuana plant contains more than 460 known compounds, of which more than 60 have the 21-carbon structure typical of cannabinoids. The only cannabinoid that is both highly psychoactive and present in large amounts, usually 1–5 percent by weight, is (-)(3,4-trans-delta-1-tetrahydrocannabinol, also known as delta-1-THC, delta-9-THC, or simply THC. A few other tetrahydrocannabinols are about as potent as delta-9-THC but present in only a few varieties of cannabis and in much smaller quantities. A number of synthetic congeners (chemical relatives) of THC have been developed under such names as synhexyl, nabilone, and levonatradol. The other two major types of cannabinoid are the cannabidiols and the cannabinols. It appears that the plant first produces the mildly active cannabidiols, which are converted to tetrahydrocannabinols and then broken down to relatively inactive cannabinols as the plant matures.

The recent discovery of nerve receptors in the brain stimulated by THC (and the cloning of the gene that gives rise to these receptors) suggests that the body produces its own version of the substance. The receptors are found mainly in the cerebral cortex, which governs higher thinking, and in the hippocampus, which is a locus of memory.[1]

A native of central Asia, cannabis may have been cultivated as long as ten thousand years ago. It was certainly cultivated in China by 4000 B.C. and in Turkestan by 3000 B.C. It has long been used as a medicine in India, China, the Middle East, Southeast Asia, South Africa, and South America. The first evidence for medicinal use of cannabis is an herbal published during the reign of the Chinese emperor Chen Nung five thousand years ago. Cannabis was recommended for malaria, constipation, rheumatic pains, "absentmindedness," and female disorders. Another Chinese herbal recommended a mixture of hemp, resin, and wine as an analgesic during surgery. In India cannabis has been recommended to quicken the mind, lower fevers, induce sleep, cure dysentery, stimulate appetite, improve digestion, relieve headaches, and cure venereal disease. In Africa it was used for dysentery, malaria, and other fevers. Today certain tribes treat snake bites with hemp or smoke it before childbirth. Hemp was also noted as a remedy by Galen and other physicians of the classical and Hellenistic eras, and it was highly valued in medieval Europe. The English clergyman Robert Burton, in his famous work *The Anatomy of Melancholy,* published in 1621, suggested the use of cannabis in the treatment of depression. The *New English Dispensatory* of 1764 recommended applying hemp roots to the skin for inflammation, a remedy that was already popular in eastern Europe. The *Edinburgh New Dispensary* of 1794 included a long description of the effects of hemp and stated that the oil was useful in the treatment of coughs, venereal disease, and urinary incontinence. A few years later Nicholas Culpeper summarized all the conditions for which cannabis was supposed to be medically useful.

1. L. A. Matsuda, S. J. Lolait, M. J. Brownstein, A. C. Young, and T. I. Bonner, "Structure of a Cannabinoid Receptor and Functional Expression of the Cloned cDNA," *Nature* 346 (Aug. 9, 1990): 561–564.

But cannabis did not come into its own in the West as a medicine until the middle of the nineteenth century. During its heyday, from 1840 to 1900, more than one hundred papers were published in the Western medical literature recommending it for various illnesses and discomforts.[2] It could almost be said that physicians of a century ago knew more about cannabis than contemporary physicians do; certainly they were more interested in exploring its therapeutic potential.

The first Western physician to take an interest in cannabis as a medicine was W. B. O'Shaughnessey, a young professor at the Medical College of Calcutta who had observed its use in India. He gave cannabis to animals, satisfied himself that it was safe, and began to use it with patients suffering from rabies, rheumatism, epilepsy, and tetanus. In a report published in 1839, he wrote that he had found tincture of hemp (a solution of cannabis in alcohol, taken orally) to be an effective analgesic. He was also impressed with its muscle relaxant properties and called it "an anticonvulsive remedy of the greatest value."[3]

O'Shaughnessey returned to England in 1842 and provided cannabis to pharmacists. Doctors in Europe and the United States soon began to prescribe it for a variety of physical conditions. Cannabis was even given to Queen Victoria by her court physician. It was listed in the United States Dispensatory in 1854 (with a warning that large doses were dangerous and that it was a powerful "narcotic"). Commercial cannabis preparations could be bought in drug stores. During the Centennial Exposition of 1876 in Philadelphia, some pharmacists carried ten pounds or more of hashish.[4]

2. T. H. Mikuriya, ed., *Marijuana: Medical Papers, 1839–1972* (Oakland: Medi-Comp, 1973).

3. W. B. O'Shaughnessey, "On the Preparations of the Indian Hemp, or Gunjah (Cannabis indica): The Effects on the Animal System in Health, and Their Utility in the Treatment of Tetanus and Other Convulsive Diseases," *Transactions of the Medical and Physical Society of Bengal* (1838–1840): 421–461.

4. E. L. Abel, *Marihuana: The First Twelve Thousand Years* (New York: Plenum, 1980).

Meanwhile, reports on cannabis accumulated in the medical literature. In 1860 Dr. R. R. M'Meens reported the findings of the Committee on Cannabis Indica to the Ohio State Medical Society.[5] After
acknowledging a debt to O'Shaughnessey, M'Meens reviewed symptoms and conditions for which Indian hemp had been found useful,
including tetanus, neuralgia, dysmenorrhea (painful menstruation),
convulsions, rheumatic and childbirth pain, asthma, postpartum psychosis, gonorrhea, and chronic bronchitis. As a hypnotic (sleep-
inducing drug) he compared it to opium: "Its effects are less intense,
and the secretions are not so much suppressed by it. Digestion is
not disturbed; the appetite rather increased; . . . The whole effect of
hemp being less violent, and producing a more natural sleep, without interfering with the actions of the internal organs, it is certainly
often preferable to opium, although it is not equal to that drug in
strength and reliability." Like O'Shaughnessey, M'Meens emphasized
the remarkable capacity of cannabis to stimulate appetite.

Interest persisted into the next generation. In 1887, H. A. Hare recommended the capacity of hemp to subdue restlessness and anxiety
and distract a patient's mind in terminal illness. In these circumstances, he wrote, "The patient, whose most painful symptom has
been mental trepidation, may become more happy or even hilarious."[6] He believed cannabis to be as effective a pain reliever as opium:
"During the time that this remarkable drug is relieving pain, a very
curious psychical condition sometimes manifests itself; namely, that
the diminution of the pain seems to be due to its fading away in the
distance, so that the pain becomes less and less, just as the pain in a
delicate ear would grow less and less as a beaten drum was carried
farther and farther out of the range of hearing."[7] Hare also noted
that hemp is an excellent topical anesthetic, especially for the mucous

5. R. R. M'Meens, "Report of the Committee on Cannabis Indica," *Transactions,*
Fifteenth Annual Meeting of the Ohio State Medical Society, Columbus, 1860.
6. H. A. Hare, "Clinical and Physiological Notes on the Action of Cannabis indica," *Therapeutic Gazette* 11 (1887): 225–226.
7. Ibid., 226.

membranes of the mouth and tongue—a property well known to dentists in the nineteenth century.

In 1890, J. R. Reynolds, a British physician, summarized thirty years of experience with Cannabis indica, recommending it for patients with "senile insomnia" and suggesting that "in this class of cases I have found nothing comparable in utility to a moderate dose of Indian hemp." According to Reynolds, hemp remained effective for months and even years without an increase in the dose. He also found it valuable in the treatment of various forms of neuralgia, including tic douloureux (a painful facial neurological disorder), and added that it was useful in preventing migraine attacks: "Very many victims of this malady have for years kept their suffering in abeyance by taking hemp at the moment of threatening or onset of the attack." He also found it useful for certain kinds of epilepsy, for depression, and sometimes for asthma and dysmenorrhea.[8]

Doctor J. B. Mattison, urging physicians to continue using hemp, in 1891 called it "a drug that has a special value in some morbid conditions and the intrinsic merit and safety of which entitles it to a place it once held in therapeutics."[9] He reviewed its uses as an analgesic and hypnotic, with special reference to dysmenorrhea, chronic rheumatism, asthma, and gastric ulcer, and added that "it has proved an efficient substitute for the poppy" in morphine addicts. One of his cases was "a naval surgeon, nine years a ten grains daily subcutaneous morphia taker . . . [who] recovered with less than a dozen doses."[10] The use of cannabis in treating drug addiction had already been reported in 1889 by E. A. Birch. He treated a chloral hydrate addict and an opiate addict with pills containing Cannabis indica and found a prompt response in both cases, with improved appetite and sound sleep.[11]

---

8. J. R. Reynolds, "Therapeutic Uses and Toxic Effects of Cannabis indica," Lancet 1 (1890): 637.

9. J. B. Mattison, "Cannabis indica as an Anodyne and Hypnotic," St. Louis Medical Surgical Journal 61 (1891): 266.

10. Ibid., 268.

11. E. A. Birch, "The Use of Indian Hemp in the Treatment of Chronic Chloral and Chronic Opium Poisoning," Lancet 1 (1889): 625.

But for Mattison the most important use of cannabis was in treating "that opprobrium of the healing art—migraine." Reviewing his own and earlier physicians' experiences, he concluded that cannabis not only blocks the pain of migraine but prevents migraine attacks.[12] Years later William Osler expressed his agreement, saying that cannabis was "probably the most satisfactory remedy" for migraine.[13]

Mattison's report concluded on a wistful note:

> Dr. Suckling wrote me: "The young men rarely prescribe it." To them I specially commend it. With a wish for speedy effect, it is so easy to use that modern mischief maker, hypodermic morphia, that they [young physicians] are prone to forget remote results of incautious opiate giving.
>
> Would that the wisdom which has come to their professional fathers through, it may be, a hapless experience might serve them to steer clear of narcotic shoals on which many a patient has gone awreck.
>
> Indian hemp is not here lauded as a specific. It will, at times, fail. So do other drugs. But the many cases in which it acts well entitle it to a large and lasting confidence.[14]

As he noted, the medical use of cannabis was already in decline by 1890. The potency of cannabis preparations was too variable, and individual responses to orally ingested cannabis seemed erratic and unpredictable. Another reason for the neglect of research on the analgesic properties of cannabis was the greatly increased use of opiates after the invention of the hypodermic syringe in the 1850s allowed soluble drugs to be injected for fast pain relief; hemp products are insoluble in water and so cannot easily be administered by injection. Toward the end of the nineteenth century, the development of such synthetic drugs as aspirin, chloral hydrate, and barbiturates, which are chemically more stable than *Cannabis indica* and therefore more

12. Mattison, "*Cannabis indica* as Anodyne," 266–267.
13. W. Osler, *The Principles and Practice of Medicine,* 8th ed. (New York: Appleton, 1913), 1089.
14. Mattison, "*Cannabis indica* as anodyne," 271.

reliable, hastened the decline of cannabis as a medicine. But the new drugs had striking disadvantages. Five hundred to a thousand people die from aspirin-induced bleeding each year in the United States, and barbiturates are, of course, far more dangerous yet. One might have expected physicians looking for better analgesics and hypnotics to have turned to cannabinoid substances, especially after 1940, when it became possible to study congeners (chemical relatives) of THC that might have more stable and specific effects.

But the Marihuana Tax Act of 1937 undermined any such experimentation. This law was the culmination of a campaign organized by the Federal Bureau of Narcotics under Harry Anslinger in which the public was led to believe that marihuana was addictive and caused violent crimes, psychosis, and mental deterioration. The film *Reefer Madness,* made as part of Anslinger's campaign, may be a joke to the sophisticated today, but it was once regarded as a serious attempt to address a social problem, and the atmosphere and attitudes it exemplified and promoted continue to influence American culture today.

Under the Marihuana Tax Act, anyone using the hemp plant for certain defined industrial or medical purposes was required to register and pay a tax of a dollar an ounce. A person using marihuana for any other purpose had to pay a tax of $100 an ounce on unregistered transactions. Those failing to comply were subject to large fines or prison terms for tax evasion. The law was not aimed at medical use of marihuana—its purpose was to discourage recreational marihuana smoking. It was put in the form of a revenue measure to evade the effect of Supreme Court decisions that reserved to the states the right to regulate most commercial transactions. By forcing some marihuana transactions to be registered and others to be taxed heavily, the government could make it prohibitively expensive to obtain the drug legally for any other than medical purposes. Almost incidentally, the law made medical use of cannabis difficult because of the extensive paperwork required of doctors who wished to use it. The Federal Bureau of Narcotics followed up with "anti-diversion" regulations that contributed to physicians' disenchantment. Cannabis was removed from the United States Pharmacopoeia and National Formulary in 1941.

A reading of the hearings in which the bill was examined by the House Ways and Means Committee before its passage shows how little data supported the judgment that marihuana was harmful and how much mass hysteria surrounded the subject. The only dissident witness was W. C. Woodward, a physician-lawyer serving as legislative counsel for the American Medical Association. He supported the aims of Congress but argued for less restrictive legislation on the grounds that future investigators might discover substantial medical uses for cannabis. In reference to marihuana "addiction," Woodward commented:

> The newspapers have called attention to it so prominently that there must be some grounds for their statements. It has surprised me, however, that the facts on which these statements have been based have not been brought before this committee by competent primary evidence. We are referred to newspaper publications concerning the prevalence of marihuana addiction. We are told that the use of marihuana causes crime.
>
> But as yet no one has been produced from the Bureau of Prisons to show the number of prisoners who have been found addicted to the marihuana habit. An informal inquiry shows that the Bureau of Prisons has no evidence on that point.
>
> You have been told that school children are great users of marihuana cigarettes. No one has been summoned from the Children's Bureau to show the nature and extent of the habit among children.
>
> Inquiry of the Children's Bureau shows that they have had no occasion to investigate it and know nothing particularly of it.
>
> Inquiry of the Office of Education—and they certainly should know something of the prevalence of the habit among the school children of the county, if there is a prevalence of the habit—indicates that they have had no occasion to investigate and know nothing of it.[15]

---

15. U.S. Congress, House Ways and Means Committee, Hearings on H.R. 6385: Taxation of Marihuana, 75th Cong., 1st sess., Apr. 27, 1937, 91, 94.

Congressmen questioned Woodward closely and critically about his educational background, his relationship to the American Medical Association, and his views on medical legislation of the previous fifteen years. His objections to the quality and sources of the evidence against cannabis did not endear him to the legislators. Representative John Dingell's questions are typical:

Mr. Dingell: We know that it is a habit that is spreading, particularly among youngsters. We learn that from the pages of the newspapers. You say that Michigan has a law regulating it. We have a State Law, but we do not seem to be able to get anywhere with it, because, as I have said, the habit is growing. The number of victims is increasing each year.

Dr. Woodward: There is no evidence of that.

Dr. Dingell: I have not been impressed by your testimony here as reflecting the sentiment of the high-class members of the medical profession in my State. I am confident that the medical profession in the State of Michigan, and in Wayne County particularly, or in my district, will subscribe wholeheartedly to any law that will suppress this thing, despite the fact that there is a $1 tax imposed.

Dr. Woodward: If there was any law that would absolutely suppress the thing, perhaps that is true, but when the law simply contains provisions that impose a useless expense, and does not accomplish the result—

Mr. Dingell (interposing): That is simply your personal opinion. That is kindred to the opinion you entertained with reference to the Harrison Narcotics Act.

Dr. Woodward: If we had been asked to cooperate in drafting it—

Mr. Dingell (interposing): You are not cooperating in drafting this at all.

Dr. Woodward: As a matter of fact, it does not serve to suppress the use of opium and cocaine.

Mr. Dingell: The medical profession should be doing its utmost to aid in the suppression of this curse that is eating the very vitals of the Nation.

Dr. Woodward: They are.

Mr. Dingell: Are you not simply piqued because you were not consulted in the drafting of the bill? [16]

Woodward was finally cut off with the admonition: "You are not cooperative in this. If you want to advise us on legislation you ought to come here with some constructive proposals rather than criticisms, rather than trying to throw obstacles in the way of something that the Federal Government is trying to do." [17] His testimony was futile. The bill became law on October 1, 1937. Many state laws, just as punitive and hastily conceived, followed.

One of the few public officials who responded rationally to the issue of marihuana in the 1930s was New York's Mayor Fiorello LaGuardia. In 1938 he appointed a committee of scientists to study the medical, sociological, and psychological aspects of marihuana use in New York City. Two internists, three psychiatrists, two pharmacologists, a public health expert, the commissioners of Correction, Health, and Hospitals, and the director of the Division of Psychiatry of the Department of Hospitals made up the committee. They began their investigations in 1940 and presented detailed findings in 1944 under the title "The Marihuana Problem in the City of New York." This largely disregarded study dispelled many of the myths that had spurred passage of the tax act. The committee found no proof that major crime was associated with marihuana or that it caused aggressive or antisocial behavior; marihuana was not sexually overstimulating and did not change personality; there was no evidence of acquired tolerance.

In September 1942 the *American Journal of Psychiatry* published "The Psychiatric Aspects of Marihuana Intoxication," by two of the study's investigators, Samuel Allentuck and Karl M. Bowman. Among other things, Allentuck and Bowman wrote that habituation to cannabis is not as strong as habituation to tobacco or alcohol. Three months later, in December, an editorial in the *Journal of the American Medical Association* described Allentuck and Bowman's article as "a care-

16. Ibid., 116.
17. Ibid., 117.

ful study" and mentioned potential therapeutic uses of cannabis in the treatment of depression, appetite loss, and opiate addiction. But in the next few years that journal's editors were induced to change their minds under government pressure. They received and published letters denouncing the LaGuardia report from Bureau of Narcotics Director Harry Anslinger in January 1943 and from R. J. Bouquet, an expert working for the Narcotics Commission of the League of Nations, in April 1944. Finally, the American Medical Association expressed its agreement with the Federal Bureau of Narcotics in the following editorial, published in April 1945:

> For many years medical scientists have considered cannabis a dangerous drug. Nevertheless, a book called *Marihuana Problems* by the New York City Mayor's Committee on Marihuana submits an analysis by seventeen doctors of tests on 77 prisoners and, on this narrow and thoroughly unscientific foundation, draws sweeping and inadequate conclusions which minimize the harmfulness of marihuana. Already the book has done harm . . . . The book states unqualifiedly to the public that the use of this narcotic does not lead to physical, mental or moral degeneration and that permanent deleterious effects from its continued use were not observed on 77 prisoners. This statement has already done great damage to the cause of law enforcement. Public officials will do well to disregard this unscientific, uncritical study, and continue to regard marihuana as a menace wherever it is purveyed.

In the words of A. S. deRopp, the journal had "abandoned its customary restraint and voiced its editorial wrath in scolding tones. So fierce was the editorial that one might suppose that the learned members of the mayor's committee . . . had formed some unhallowed league with the 'tea-pad' proprietors [owners of places where marihuana users gathered to smoke] to undermine the city's health by deliberately misrepresenting the facts about marihuana."[18] For more

18. S. Allentuck and K. M. Bowman, "The Psychiatric Aspects of Marihuana Intoxication," *American Journal of Psychiatry* 99 (1942): 248–251; Editorial: Recent Inves-

than forty years after that editorial, the American Medical Association steadfastly maintained a position on marihuana closely allied to that of the Federal Bureau of Narcotics and its successor agencies.

Although virtually no medical investigation of cannabis was conducted for many years, the government did not entirely lose interest. Shortly after one of us (L.G.) published a book on marihuana in 1971, a chemist who had read it told us that his employer, the Arthur D. Little Company, had been given millions of dollars in government contracts to identify military uses for cannabis. He said they had found none but had come across important therapeutic leads. He visited us to discuss the economic feasibility of developing cannabinoid congeners commercially, but he could not give us the evidence because it was classified.

In the 1960s, as large numbers of people began to use marihuana recreationally, anecdotes about its medical utility began to appear, generally not in the medical literature but in the form of letters to popular magazines like *Playboy*. Meanwhile, legislative concern about recreational use increased, and in 1970 Congress passed the Controlled Substances Act. This law assigned psychoactive drugs to five schedules and placed cannabis in Schedule I, the most restrictive. According to the legal definition, Schedule I drugs have no medical use and a high potential for abuse, and they cannot be used safely even under a doctor's supervision. By that time the renaissance of interest in cannabis as a medicine was already well under way. Two years later, in 1972, the National Organization for the Reform of Marihuana Laws (NORML) petitioned the Bureau of Narcotics and Dangerous Drugs (formerly the Federal Bureau of Narcotics) to transfer marihuana to Schedule II so that it could be legally prescribed by physicians. As the legal proceedings have continued, other parties have joined, including the Drug Policy Foundation and the Physicians Association for AIDS Care.

---

tigation of Marihuana, *Journal of the American Medical Association* (hereafter *JAMA*) 120 (1942): 1128–1129; Letter: Anslinger, "The Psychiatric Aspects of Marihuana Intoxication," *JAMA* 121 (1943): 212–213; Letter: Bouquet, "Marihuana Intoxication," *JAMA* 124 (1944): 1010–1011; Editorial: "Marihuana Problems," *JAMA* 127 (1945): 1129; R. S. deRopp, *Drugs and the Mind* (New York: St. Martin's, 1957), 108–109.

The hearings before the Bureau of Narcotics and Dangerous Drugs (BNDD) were instructive. As one of us (L.G.) waited to testify on the medical uses of cannabis, he witnessed the effort to place pentazocine (Talwin ®), a synthetic opioid analgesic made by Winthrop Pharmaceuticals, on the schedule of dangerous drugs. The testimony indicated several hundred cases of addiction, a number of deaths from overdose, and considerable evidence of abuse. Six lawyers from the drug company, briefcases in hand, came forward to prevent the classification of pentazocine or at least to ensure that it was placed in one of the less restrictive schedules. They succeeded in part; it became a Schedule IV drug. In the testimony on cannabis, the next drug to be considered, there was no evidence of overdose deaths or addiction—simply many witnesses, both patients and physicians, who testified to its medical utility. The government refused to transfer it to Schedule II. Might the outcome have been different if a large drug company with enormous financial resources had a commercial interest in cannabis?

In rejecting the NORML petition, the Bureau of Narcotics and Dangerous Drugs failed to call for public hearings as required by law. The reason it gave was that reclassification would violate U.S. treaty obligations under the United Nations Single Convention on Narcotic Substances. NORML responded in January 1974 by filing a suit against the BNDD. The U.S. Second Circuit Court of Appeals reversed the bureau's dismissal of the petition, remanding the case for reconsideration and criticizing both the bureau and the Department of Justice. In September 1975, the Drug Enforcement Administration (DEA), successor to the BNDD, acknowledged that treaty obligations did not prevent the rescheduling of marihuana but continued to refuse public hearings. NORML again filed suit. In October 1980, after much further legal maneuvering, the Court of Appeals remanded the NORML petition to the DEA for reconsideration for the third time. The government reclassified synthetic THC as a Schedule II drug in 1985 but kept marihuana itself—and THC derived from marihuana—in Schedule I. Finally, in May 1986, the DEA administrator announced the public hearings ordered by the court seven years earlier.

Those hearings began in the summer of 1986 and lasted two years.

The parties who sought rescheduling were NORML, a membership-funded educational organization, founded in 1970, which opposes all criminal prohibitions against marihuana and marihuana smoking; the Alliance for Cannabis Therapeutics, a nonprofit organization founded in 1980 to make marihuana available by prescription; the Cannabis Corporation of America, a pharmaceutical firm established with the intention of extracting natural cannabinoids for therapeutic use when cannabis is placed in Schedule II; and the Ethiopian Zion Coptic Church, which considers marihuana a sacred plant essential to its religious rituals. These groups were opposed by the DEA, the International Chiefs of Police, and the National Federation of Parents for Drug-Free Youth, another membership-funded educational organization.

The lengthy hearings involved many witnesses, including both patients and doctors, and thousands of pages of documentation. The record of these hearings constitutes the most extensive contemporary exploration of the evidence on cannabis as a medicine. Administrative law judge Francis J. Young reviewed the evidence and rendered his decision on September 6, 1988. Young said that approval by a "significant minority" of physicians was enough to meet the standard of "currently accepted medical use in treatment in the United States" established by the Controlled Substances Act for a Schedule II drug. He added that "marijuana, in its natural form, is one of the safest therapeutically active substances known to man . . . . One must reasonably conclude that there is accepted safety for use of marijuana under medical supervision. To conclude otherwise, on the record, would be unreasonable, arbitrary, and capricious." Young went on to recommend "that the Administrator [of the DEA] conclude that the marijuana plant considered as a whole has a currently accepted medical use in treatment in the United States, that there is no lack of accepted safety for use of it under medical supervision and that it may lawfully be transferred from Schedule I to Schedule II."[19]

19. Drug Enforcement Agency (hereafter DEA), In the Matter of Marijuana Rescheduling Petition, Docket 86–22, Opinion, Recommended Ruling, Findings of Fact, Conclusions of Law, and Decision of Administrative Law Judge, Sept. 6, 1988.

In determining what "currently accepted medical use" meant for legal purposes, Judge Young was adopting the view of the petitioners and rejecting that of the DEA, whose criteria were the result of a previous legal challenge involving the drug 3,4-methylenedioxymethamphetamine (MDMA). In 1984 the DEA placed this previously unscheduled drug in Schedule I. The placement was challenged by a group of physicians and others who believed that MDMA had therapeutic potential. After extensive hearings, the administrative law judge rejected the DEA's position that MDMA had no accepted medical use in treatment in the United States, and agreed with the challengers that it should be placed in Schedule III rather than Schedule I. The DEA administrator rejected this recommendation. The challengers appealed to the U.S. First Circuit Court of Appeals, which ruled in their favor, finding that formal approval for marketing by the Food and Drug Administration, the DEA's criterion for "accepted medical use in treatment in the United States," was unacceptable under the terms of the Controlled Substances Act.[20]

The DEA administrator responded with the following new criteria for accepted medical use of a drug: (1) scientifically determined and accepted knowledge of its chemistry; (2) scientific knowledge of its toxicology and pharmacology in animals; (3) effectiveness in human beings established through scientifically designed clinical trials; (4) general availability of the substance and information about its use; (5) recognition of its clinical use in generally accepted pharmacopoeia, medical references, journals, or textbooks; (6) specific indications for the treatment of recognized disorders; (7) recognition of its use by organizations or associations of physicians; and (8) recognition and use by a substantial segment of medical practitioners in the United States. These were the criteria rejected by Judge Young in his marihuana decision.

The DEA disregarded the opinion of its own administrative law judge and refused to reschedule marihuana. The agency's lawyer remarked, "The judge seems to hang his hat on what he calls a re-

20. Grinspoon v. DEA, 828 F.2d 881 (1st Cir. 1987).

spectable minority of physicians. What percent are you talking about? One half of one percent? One quarter of one percent?" DEA Administrator John Lawn went further, calling claims for the medical utility of marihuana a "dangerous and cruel hoax."[21] In March 1991 the plaintiffs appealed yet again, and in April the District of Columbia Court of Appeals unanimously ordered the DEA to reexamine its standards, suggesting that they were illogical and that marihuana could never satisfy them. An illegal drug could not be used by a substantial number of doctors or cited as a remedy in medical texts. As the court pointed out, "We are hard pressed to understand how one could show that any Schedule I drug was in general use or generally available."[22] The court returned the case to the DEA for further explanation, but it offered no direct challenge to the central dogma that marihuana lacks therapeutic value. The DEA issued a final rejection of all pleas for reclassification in March 1992.

In spite of the obstructionism of the federal government, a few patients have been able to obtain marihuana legally for therapeutic purposes. State governments began to respond in a limited way to pressure from patients and physicians in the 1970s. In 1978, New Mexico enacted the first law designed to make marihuana available for medical use. Thirty-three states followed in the late 1970s and early 1980s.[23] In 1992, Massachusetts became the thirty-fifth to enact such legislation.

But the laws proved difficult to implement. Since marihuana is not recognized as a medicine under federal law, states could dispense it only by establishing formal research programs and getting FDA approval for an IND (Investigational New Drug) application.

21. Marijuana Scheduling Petition, Denial of Petition, *Federal Register* 54, no. 249 (Dec. 29, 1988), 53784.
22. U.S. Court of Appeals, District of Columbia Circuit, Docket 90–1019, Petition for Review of Orders of the DEA, Apr. 26, 1991, 9.
23. Alabama, Alaska, Arizona, Arkansas, California, Colorado, Connecticut, Florida, Georgia, Illinois, Iowa, Louisiana, Maine, Michigan, Minnesota, Montana, Nevada, New Hampshire, New Jersey, New York, North Carolina, Ohio, Oklahoma, Oregon, Rhode Island, South Carolina, Tennessee, Texas, Vermont, Virginia, Washington, West Virginia, and Wisconsin.

Many states gave up as soon as the officials in charge of the programs confronted the regulatory nightmare of the relevant federal laws. Nevertheless, between 1978 and 1984, seventeen states received permission to establish programs for the use of marihuana in treating glaucoma and the nausea induced by cancer chemotherapy. Each of these programs has fallen into abeyance because of the many problems involved.

Take the case of Louisiana, where a law was passed in 1978 establishing a program that allowed a Marihuana Prescription Board to review and approve applications by physicians to treat patients with cannabis. The board would have preferred a simple procedure in which medical decisions would be entrusted to the practicing physician, but federal agencies would not supply cannabis without an IND. That would have required an enormous amount of paperwork and would have made the program intolerably cumbersome. The board therefore decided to use an approved research program operated by the National Cancer Institute, which was limited to cancer patients and employed only synthetic THC. Marihuana itself was not made legally available to any patient in Louisiana. With these limitations, the program proved ineffective. Patients felt compelled to use illicit cannabis, and at least one was arrested.[24]

Only ten states eventually established programs in which cannabis was used as a medicine. Among these New Mexico was the first and the most successful, largely because of the efforts of a young cancer patient, Lynn Pierson. In 1978 the state legislature enacted a law allowing physicians to prescribe marihuana to patients suffering from the nausea and vomiting of cancer chemotherapy. The law was later modified to comply with federal IND regulations requiring a research program. Considerable friction immediately developed between the FDA and the people in charge of the New Mexico program. The FDA demanded studies with placebos (inactive substances) as controls;

---

24. DEA, Marijuana Rescheduling Petition, Docket 86–22, Affidavit of Philip Jobe, Ph.D.

the physicians in the New Mexico program wanted to provide sick patients with care. The FDA wanted to proceed slowly; the attitudes of the physicians reflected the urgency of their patients' needs. Eventually a compromise was reached. Patients would be assigned at random to treatment with marihuana cigarettes or synthetic THC capsules. But prolonged delays suggested to the New Mexico officials that the FDA was not dealing in good faith, and tensions began to grow. At one point state officials even considered using confiscated marihuana, and the Chief of the State Highway Patrol was asked whether it could be supplied.

In August 1978, Lynn Pierson, who had made such a heroic effort to establish a compassionate program, died of cancer without ever having received legal marihuana. Now the FDA approved the New Mexico IND, only to rescind the approval a few weeks later, after the public furor surrounding Pierson's death had died down. At that point New Mexico officials considered holding a public press conference to condemn federal officials for "unethical and immoral behavior." Finally, in November 1978, the program was approved; supplies of marihuana were promised within a month, but not delivered for two months.

The random design of the program was soon violated. Patients discussed among themselves the relative merits of the two types of treatment and switched when they wanted; this also gave them a sense of control over their own care. But many believed, despite the denials of the National Institute of Drug Abuse (NIDA), that the cigarettes they received were not of adequate potency. The state never conducted an independent assay. Some patients left the program in order to buy cannabis on the streets, saying it was better than either government marihuana or synthetic THC.

From 1978 to 1986 about 250 cancer patients in New Mexico received either marihuana or THC after conventional medications failed to control their nausea and vomiting. For these patients both marihuana and THC were effective, but marihuana was superior. More than 90 percent reported significant or total relief from nausea and vomiting. Only three adverse effects were reported in the entire program—anxiety reactions that were easily treated by simple reassurance.[25]

The successful programs in other states resembled the one in New Mexico. It was understood that "research" was merely a disguise; the aim was to relieve suffering. Although the results did not meet the methodological standards for controlled clinical research, they did confirm the effectiveness of cannabis and the advantage of smoked marihuana over oral THC. Incidentally, none of the programs reported problems with abuse or diversion of either THC or marihuana cigarettes.

A New York State Department of Health report on the therapeutic use of cannabis asked why more patients and physicians had not enrolled in the New York Program. It concluded that there were several reasons. First, physicians were skeptical because of their limited training and experience. Second, bureaucratic obstacles were enormous. As the report states, "Hospital pharmacists and administrators complain about paperwork and procedures. Physicians complain about burdensome reporting and application requirements. At least 16 physicians have inquired into the availability of marijuana, but have chosen not to enroll in the program because they perceive a large amount of bureaucratic procedure." A third possibility was that many patients and physicians decided it was easier to get marihuana of good quality on the street.[26]

At about the same time the state programs were being instituted, growing demand forced the FDA to institute an Individual Treatment IND (commonly referred to as Compassionate Use IND or Compassionate IND) for the use of individual physicians whose patients needed marihuana. The application process was not easy, because INDs were designed for an entirely different purpose—making

25. Ibid., Affidavit of Daniel Danzak, M.D.

26. *Annual Report to the Governor and Legislature on the Antonio G. Olivieri Controlled Substances Therapeutic Research Program,* New York State Department of Health, Sept. 1, 1982.

pharmaceutical companies assure the safety of new drugs. First the patient in need of cannabis had to persuade a physician to apply to the FDA for an IND. The physician then had to file a special form with the DEA covering Schedule I drugs. If the application was approved by both agencies, the physician then had to fill out special order forms for marihuana, which were sent to the National Institute of Drug Abuse (NIDA). NIDA grew cannabis on a farm at the University of Mississippi—the only legal marihuana farm in the United States—and sent it to North Carolina, where it was rolled into cigarettes that were supposed to have the same potency as street marihuana (2 percent THC). NIDA then shipped the marihuana to a designated pharmacy that had to comply with stringent DEA regulations for drug security. The application process took four to eight months. Both the FDA and the DEA required constant prodding and rarely responded within the time specified by law. According to the Alliance for Cannabis Therapeutics, which helped a number of patients and physicians through the process, government agencies routinely seemed to lose some of the application forms, and the doctor had to resubmit them, sometimes more than once. Understandably, most physicians did not want to become entangled in the paperwork, especially since many also believe there is some stigma attached to prescribing cannabis.

In 1976 Robert Randall became the first patient to receive a Compassionate IND for the use of marihuana. In the next 13 years the government reluctantly awarded about a half dozen more. Then, in 1989, the FDA was deluged with applications from people with AIDS. A case that called attention to the absurd and appalling consequences of the medical ban on marihuana was the government assault on Kenneth and Barbra Jenks, a Florida couple in their twenties who contracted AIDS through a blood transfusion given to the husband, a hemophiliac. Both were suffering from nausea, vomiting, and appetite loss caused by AIDS or AZT; their doctor feared that Barbra Jenks would die of starvation before the disease killed her. In early 1989 the Jenks learned about marihuana through a support group for people with AIDS. They began to smoke it and for a year they led a fairly normal life. They felt better, regained lost weight and were able to stay out of the hospital; Kenneth Jenks even kept his full-time job.

Then someone informed on them. On March 29, 1990, ten armed narcotics officers battered down the door of their trailer home, held a gun to Barbra Jenks' head, and seized the evidence of crime, two small marihuana plants they had been growing because they could not afford to pay the street price of the drug. Cultivation of marihuana is a felony in Florida; the Jenkses faced up to five years in prison. At their trial in July the Jenkses used the defense of medical necessity, which is rarely successful. The judge rejected this defense and convicted the Jenkses, although he imposed no real punishment. The conviction was later overturned by a higher court and the defense of medical necessity sustained.

The case received national publicity and the Jenkses were able to obtain a Compassionate IND. Now the FDA was inundated with new requests from AIDS sufferers. The number of extant Compassionate INDs rose from five to thirty-four in a year. In early June 1991, Deputy National Drug Control Policy Director Herbert D. Kleber assured a national television audience that anyone with a legitimate medical need for marihuana would be able to get a Compassionate IND. But a few weeks later, on June 21, James O. Mason, chief of the Public Health Service, announced that the program would be suspended because it undercut the administration's opposition to the use of illegal drugs. "If it is perceived that the Public Health Service is going around giving marihuana to folks, there would be a perception that this stuff can't be so bad," Mason said. "It gives a bad signal. I don't mind doing that if there is no other way of helping these people . . . . But there is not a shred of evidence that smoking marihuana assists a person with AIDS." Since then, no new Compassionate INDs have been granted, despite hundreds of applications.

After keeping the program in limbo "under review" for nine months, the Public Health Service discontinued it in March 1992. Twenty-eight patients whose applications have already been approved (including some whose stories follow) will not be supplied with the promised marihuana. Nine patients now receiving marihuana will continue to receive it. After more than twenty years in which hundreds of people have worked through state legislatures, federal courts, and administrative agencies to make marihuana available for suffering people, these nine are the only ones for whom it is not still a forbidden medicine.

2 Cannabis as a Medicine

In our century cannabis has been proposed or shown to be useful as a medicine for many disorders and symptoms. These uses range from the proven to the speculative, but they should all be of interest to anyone concerned about human suffering. The narratives of patients illustrate most vividly not only marihuana's therapeutic properties but also the unnecessary further pain and anxiety imposed on sick people who must obtain it illegally.

CANCER CHEMOTHERAPY

Chemotherapy is one of the most important cancer treatments developed in the past several decades. Administered intravenously once every few weeks, chemotherapeutic agents are among the most powerful and toxic chemicals used in medicine. In attacking cancer cells, they also kill healthy body cells, producing extremely unpleasant and dangerous side effects. Among the most widely used chemotherapeutic agents are cisplatin (Platinol®), doxorubicin (Adriamycin®), cyclophosphamide (Cytoxan®), ifosfamide (Ifex®), and nitrogen mustard derivatives, including such drugs as melphalan (Alkeran®) and chlorambucil (Leukeran®).

Cisplatin can cause deafness or life-threatening kidney failure. Ifosfamide may cause bleeding and bruising; cyclophosphamide suppresses the immune system; doxorubicin can destroy heart muscle. Nitrogen mustard derivatives are so toxic that they eat away the skin or any other tissue they touch. If the intravenous needle through which they are being delivered leaks or slips out of the vein, the resulting scar tissue may cause the patient to lose the use of an arm. Most of these drugs also cause hair loss, and any of them may cause a second type of cancer while suppressing the original disease. Doses must be carefully calculated to prevent kidney, heart, or respiratory failure.

But the most common, and for many patients the most troublesome, side effect of these drugs is profound nausea and vomiting. Retching (dry heaves) may last for hours or even days after each treatment, followed by days and even weeks of nausea. Patients may break bones or rupture the esophagus while vomiting. The sense of a loss of control can be emotionally devastating. Furthermore, many patients eat almost nothing because they cannot stand the sight or smell of food. As they lose weight and strength, they find it more and more difficult to sustain the will to live.

Patients become more apprehensive with each successive treatment. Some develop a conditioned reaction that causes them to vomit when they walk into the treatment room, or even before they arrive at the hospital. A few have been known to vomit reflexively on seeing a member of the treatment team on the street. If the nausea and vomiting cannot be controlled, the patient's complaints may cause doctors to lower the dose and jeopardize the effectiveness of the therapy. For many patients, the side effects of chemotherapy seem worse than the cancer itself, and they discontinue treatment, not only to eliminate the discomfort but also to regain control over their lives. Some insist on stopping even though they know it means certain death. In otherwise treatable patients who refuse therapy, the nausea and vomiting should be considered a potentially lethal form of toxicity.

Many patients, fortunately, obtain sufficient relief from such standard antiemetic drugs as prochlorperazine (Compazine®) or the newer ondansetron (Zofran®). But in some cases these drugs never work or soon stop working. Zofran is now considered the most effective of the standard antiemetics, but it must be administered over a period of hours through an intravenous drip while the patient remains in a hospital bed, at a cost of hundreds of dollars per treatment. As the results of the state research programs discussed above indicate, marihuana may be a remarkably effective substitute for standard drugs. In one study of fifty-six patients who got no relief from standard antiemetic agents, 78 percent became symptom-free when they smoked marihuana.[1]

One of us (L.G.) has had a personal encounter with this therapeutic effect:

Early in 1972, after the death of Sidney Farber, the Harvard child oncologist for whom the Sidney Farber Cancer Research Center was named, my wife and I were invited to dinner at the home of a fellow Harvard Medical School faculty member. He wanted me to meet Emil Frei, who had arrived from Houston to serve as Dr. Farber's successor.

At dinner, Dr. Frei told me about an eighteen-year-old Houston man with leukemia who had become more and more resistant to cancer chemotherapy because he could no longer tolerate the nausea and vomiting. His doctors and his family were finding it increasingly difficult to persuade him to take the drug on which his life depended.

One day, to Dr. Frei's surprise, the young man willingly agreed to take the drug and from then on offered no resistance to chemotherapy. He eventually revealed that he had been smoking marihuana twenty minutes before each session; it prevented all vomiting and even the slightest hint of nausea. Dr. Frei asked me whether this property was mentioned in the nineteenth-century medical literature on cannabis, and I told him that it was. On the way home my wife, Betsy, who had listened with great interest, suggested that we obtain some cannabis for our son, Danny.

1. V. Vinciguerra, T. Moore, and E. Brennan, "Inhalation Marijuana as an Antiemetic for Cancer Chemotherapy," *New York State Journal of Medicine* 88 (October 1988): 525–527.

Danny was first given the diagnosis of acute lymphatic leukemia in July 1967; he was ten years old. For the first few years he was good-natured about his treatment at Children's Hospital in Boston, and even about the occasional need for hospitalization. But in 1971 he started taking the first of the drugs that cause severe nausea and vomiting.

Danny was one of those patients in whom these reactions were uncontrollable and not sufficiently alleviated by standard antiemetics. He would start to vomit shortly after treatment and continue retching for up to eight hours. He vomited in the car as we drove home, and on arriving he had to lie in bed with his head over a bucket on the floor. Still, I was shocked when Betsy suggested that we find cannabis for Danny. I objected because it was against the law and because it might embarrass staff members at the hospital, who had been so remarkable in their commitment to Danny's care. I dismissed the idea.

Danny's next treatment was two weeks later. When I arrived, Betsy and Danny were already in the treatment room. I shall never forget my surprise. Normally my wife and son were in a state of great anxiety before the treatment began, but this time they were completely relaxed, and, what is more, seemed almost to be playing a joke on me.

Finally, they let me in on the secret. On the way to the clinic that morning they had stopped near Wellesley High School, and Betsy had asked one of Danny's friends to get her some marihuana. Once he recovered from his disbelief, the friend had run off and reappeared a few minutes later with a small amount of marihuana. Betsy and Danny had smoked it in the parking lot of the hospital just before entering the clinic.

My surprise gave way to relief as I saw how comfortable Danny was. He did not protest as he was given the medicine, and we were all delighted when no nausea or vomiting followed. On the way home he asked his mother if he could stop for a submarine sandwich, and when he got home he began his usual activities instead of going straight to bed. We could scarcely believe it.

The next day I called Dr. Norman Jaffe, the physician who was in charge of Danny's care. I explained what had happened and said that while I did not want to embarrass him or the rest of the medical staff, I could not forbid Danny to smoke marihuana before his next treatment. Dr. Jaffe responded by suggesting that Danny smoke marihuana in his presence in the treatment room.

Danny did that the next time. When he was given the chemotherapeutic agent, Dr. Jaffe could observe for himself that he was completely relaxed. Afterward he again asked for a submarine sandwich. From then on he used marihuana before every treatment, and we were all much more comfortable during the remaining year of his life.

Doctor Jaffe asked me to join him in reporting our observations to Dr. Frei, who was sufficiently interested to perform the first clinical experiment on the use of cannabis in cancer chemotherapy. [S. E. Sallan, N. E. Zinberg, and E. Frei III, "Antiemetic Effect of Delta-9-tetrahydracannabinol in Patients Receiving Cancer Chemotherapy," *New Eng. J. Med.* 293 (1975):795–797.]

Arnold and Mae Nutt, now in their seventies, raised three sons in Beaverton, Michigan. In 1963, shortly after his fifth birthday, Dana, the middle child, was found to have bone cancer. After surgery he received chemotherapy and radiation treatments for three months. The treatments made him very ill but did not halt the spread of the cancer, and he died in 1967. For years, the Nutts struggled to recover from their grief and the financial burden imposed by their son's illness. Then, in 1978, their oldest son, Keith, developed testicular cancer at the age of twenty-two. Mae Nutt tells his story:

Surgeons operated on Keith, removing the diseased testicle and a large number of lymph nodes. They believed they had cut out all of the cancer. Keith made a determined effort to remain active. He resumed working, and all appeared to be going well, but nine months later he discovered that his other testicle was hard and enlarged. Surgeons immediately removed it, and he was told that he would require extensive chemotherapy as well. He was given cisplatin, a new, highly toxic drug that made him extremely ill.

He would vomit violently for eight to ten hours, and afterward was so profoundly nauseated that he could not bear to look at or smell food. Compazine and other antiemetic drugs provided no noticeable relief.

In less than two months our son lost at least thirty pounds. He began to vomit bile. When there was nothing to vomit, he would simply retch and convulse. It was horrible for us to watch our child suffer such anguish from the disease and the treatment. At one point Keith told me he did not want to become like his deceased brother Dana—so sick he could not take care of himself, completely incapacitated, and a burden on the rest of the family. He told me that when things got that bad, he wanted to be able to kill himself. He made me promise that when there was no hope, I would help him end his life.

One evening I read a newspaper article about a cancer patient who had received a brown bag of marihuana on his doorstep. The article noted that medical evidence suggested it could reduce the severe nausea and vomiting caused by many anticancer therapies. The idea that marihuana had medical uses was new to my husband and me. At first I laughed at the story. It seemed unlikely that marihuana would just suddenly appear on someone's doorstep.

As a parent I was strongly opposed to marihuana and other illegal drugs. My husband and I made sure our sons knew exactly how we felt. We do not doubt that they may have experimented with marihuana while growing up, but we are also sure they had no drug problems and no illusions about our stern opposition to drug use. It was hard to believe that an illegal drug could be of any help. If marihuana had medical value, we thought that the government would know and would make it legally available by prescription.

But we were desperate, so we told Keith what we had read. He replied that other patients in the hospital who were receiving chemotherapy smoked marihuana to reduce the side effects and said it worked. We proceeded to contact our state representative, Robert Young, and asked him whether we could legally obtain marihuana for Keith. We were surprised to learn that a bill to legalize marihuana for the treatment of glaucoma and cancer was scheduled to come before the Michigan legislature. Representative Young also put us in touch with Mr. Roger Winthrop, a man who was working on the legislation with representatives and senators. He provided information on the medical uses of marihuana and told us that physicians and patients in several states had already succeeded in getting them to pass laws making it available to seriously ill patients like Keith.

Shortly after my husband and I read these materials, Keith had another round of chemotherapy, and, as always, it made him dreadfully sick. We could not stand by and watch him suffer, but, as an older couple, we did not have the slightest idea where to find marihuana. In desperation, we asked a close friend for help, an ordained Presbyterian minister who worked with local youth groups. Several days later he appeared at our door with some marihuana. It was the first time we had ever seen any.

The next day we took the marihuana to Keith in the hospital. After he smoked it his vomiting abruptly stopped. The sudden change was amazing to see. Marihuana also put an end to his nausea. When he smoked it he was constantly hungry and actually began to put on weight. His mental outlook also underwent a startling improvement. Before he started to smoke marihuana, Keith would come home from chemotherapy, shut himself in his bedroom, stuff towels under the door to keep out the smell of dinner cooking, and remain in his room or the bathroom vomiting all evening. The cancer and chemotherapy made him act like a wounded animal, timid and retiring. He had intense hot and cold flashes. His joints became swollen and painful. His hair fell out and he felt sick all over. Large pieces of skin came off at the place where the injections were given.

Smoking marihuana dramatically changed his life. Immediately before the chemotherapy he smoked one marihuana cigarette, and afterward, if he felt queasy, all or part of a second. When we arrived home he stayed in the living room and talked with his brother and father. He joined the family for dinner and ate more than his share. He became outgoing and talkative, part of our family again. He never once experienced an adverse effect. Marihuana was the safest, most benign drug he received in the course of his battle against cancer.

We made certain that all of his doctors and nurses were aware of the situation; none objected and some clearly approved. We even arranged for him to smoke marihuana in his hospital room. In effect, reasonable people caring for Keith decided that the law did not match the reality of his needs.

We learned that many cancer patients were smoking marihuana and most told their doctors, who approved but were not willing to say in public what they told their patients in their offices.

My husband and I came to resent the fact that Keith's therapy was illegal. We felt like criminals. We are honest, simple people and hate having to sneak around. We were uncomfortable asking our closest friends, our minister, and our other son, Marc, to risk arrest in order to provide Keith with the medicine he so obviously needed. We were also concerned about other parents who might not know that marihuana could help end their child's misery. We asked Keith whether we could tell his story to a local newspaper, the *Bay City Times,* to help other cancer patients. He agreed on the condition that we not supply details about the nature of his cancer and the surgical removal of his testes. As a young man in his twenties, he wanted at least that much of his life to remain private.

On the day the article about Keith appeared in the newspaper, we went to Lansing to testify before the Michigan Senate Judiciary Committee on the medical marihuana legislation. The hearings generated considerable publicity, and we began to receive phone calls from other cancer patients in Michigan and throughout the United States. Keith often spoke with them late into the night. Cancer patients and their relatives asked him for help and advice on how to smoke properly, how much to use, and how often. He even went on "house calls" several times to show patients how to roll the cigarettes or inhale the smoke. This opportunity to help others gave Keith great joy.

One day shortly after the hearings we found a small brown bag of marihuana in our mailbox. There was no note, no identification, just an ounce of marihuana. I remembered the newspaper story I had laughed at, the one in which marihuana appeared on someone's doorstep. Soon we received more marihuana in the mail. The donors usually remained anonymous, but not always. An Episcopal priest, for example, brought marihuana to our house and said he thought we would know who might benefit from it. As news spread through the grapevine, we heard from some familiar folks. One day we received a call from a woman who had attended elementary school with Arnold, my husband. She invited us to her home and offered us a cigar box filled with marihuana. She explained that her husband, recently deceased, had smoked it to help control terminal cancer pain. She had no use for it now but did not want to throw it away.

When my husband and I returned to Lansing for additional legislative hearings, Keith was back in the hospital and his cancer was spreading again. This time we were joined by another family, the Negens, of Grand Rapids, who had testified at the previous hearing without giving their names. Their daughter Deborah, twenty-one, was receiving chemotherapy for leukemia, and marihuana was the only drug that relieved the debilitating side effects. The Reverend Negen is pastor of the very conservative Dutch Christian Reform Church in Grand Rapids. He testified that he had prayed for guidance and realized that if using marihuana to help his daughter offended his congregation, he would have to leave his church. He spoke movingly about having to send his own young sons into the streets of Grand Rapids to buy marihuana for his daughter. It was easy for us to understand the Reverend Negen's distress. Like us, he was being forced to break the law to provide for his child's medical needs.

Deborah Negen herself was even more eloquent and moving as

she pleaded with the committee to consider that other seriously ill people were suffering needlessly.

On October 10, 1979, the Michigan House voted 100 to 0 in favor of making marihuana available to patients like Keith. Five days later, on October 15, the Senate concurred, 33 to 1. On the evening of Sunday, October 21, my husband and I told Keith that the Michigan Marihuana as Medicine Bill would be signed into law the next day. Keith was happy that his efforts had made a difference. He smiled and said good night. Early in the next morning he died, and later that day the bill was signed into law.

Six months after they were married in 1969, Mona Taft's husband, Harris, noticed a lump on his neck. A biopsy performed at the Massachusetts General Hospital in Boston revealed Hodgkin's disease, a malignancy of the lymph nodes. Mona Taft tells their story:

> At the time of diagnosis, Harris was gravely ill, but not yet showing the advanced, manifest symptoms of Hodgkin's disease. He immediately underwent the first of many surgical procedures: his spleen and affected lymph glands were removed through an incision that ran from his pelvic bone to his chest. As soon as the wound healed and he recovered some of his strength, he began to receive the first in what was to be a decade of anticancer treatments.
>
> Despite doctors' warnings, we were totally unprepared for the devastating effects of chemotherapy. Within ninety minutes after receiving his first chemotherapy treatment, my husband began to vomit, and the vomiting persisted for endless hours. When there was nothing left to throw up, he would get the dry heaves. A day later the vomiting would subside, but he remained so nauseated that he could not eat or even stand the sight or smell of food. The doctors prescribed a series of antiemetic drugs like Compazine. None of them worked. Harris received chemotherapy at least once a month for nearly a year. It seemed to help suppress his cancer, but it also took a terrible toll on the quality of his life.
>
> In the next seven years Harris was in and out of remission

several times. Each time the cancer returned, it was more wide-spread, the drugs used to fight it were more toxic, and the adverse reactions became more severe. Meanwhile, Harris underwent many more surgical procedures, including the removal of cancerous tissue that had spread to his brain. Later he began to find walking difficult because of cancerous tissue in his spine that was pinching the nerves leading to his legs. These tumors, too, were surgically removed. As the disease continued to spread, Harris underwent exploratory abdominal surgery; the doctors found too much cancer to remove. More chemotherapy was recommended, and radiation treatments were added, causing further nausea. Each day was becoming more and more painful for him.

One day in 1977, when we arrived at the treatment room where Harris was to receive the injection, he bolted and ran down the corridor. I found him a bit later, wandering the halls. He told me he couldn't take any more chemotherapy. He was at wit's end, exhausted by the disease, terrified by the effects of the drugs that were supposed to prolong his life. I have never before or since seen a man so genuinely and deeply frightened. Harris had come to fear the treatments more than the cancer and, he admitted, more than death itself. He told me he would choose dying over further chemotherapy.

One of the nurse practitioners overheard us and interrupted; she said she understood our problem and suggested that Harris smoke marihuana to relieve the nausea and vomiting. We were startled. Although Harris had occasionally smoked marihuana socially, he couldn't believe it would help. We asked Harris's doctor about marihuana, and he said that he couldn't encourage us to do anything illegal, but many of his younger patients were smoking marihuana and it seemed to reduce their trouble with nausea and vomiting. The message was pretty clear: Try marihuana and see if it helps. Harris had a strong will to live and, as he said, nothing to lose, so he decided to give chemotherapy one more chance and smoke some marihuana beforehand. I did not have much hope.

When Harris went for his next chemotherapy session, he was so frightened he forgot to bring his marihuana; I had to take it to him after he called from his hospital room. Doctors, nurses, and orderlies must have seen him smoking it, but no one said anything. It was as if we had all reached an unspoken understanding. After the chemotherapy I decided to stay with Harris through the night in case he needed my help. But this time there was no vomiting; he slept like a baby. It was his first full night of restful sleep in nearly seven years of anticancer treatments. The next morning he actually ate breakfast, a real breakthrough. No vomiting. No nausea. And he actually wanted to eat! I cannot describe how relieved and excited we were. Why hadn't someone told us sooner? Why had my husband gone through all those years of needless suffering?

Usually Harris was sick for weeks after receiving chemotherapy; this time he was ready to go back to work in forty-eight hours. From that time on he smoked marihuana whenever he had chemotherapy. The results were dramatic. He started to regain lost weight, and his mood improved remarkably. He became more active and outgoing, and we began to do things together that I thought we would never be able to do again. It was clear that his doctors knew what he was doing and approved; they couldn't help noticing the sudden improvement in his condition.

It is impossible for me to adequately describe what a profound difference marihuana made. Before using marihuana, Harris felt ill all the time, could not eat, could not even stand the smell of food cooking. Afterward, he remained active, ate regular meals, and could be himself. His mood, his manner, and his overall outlook were transformed. And of course, marihuana prolonged his life by allowing him to continue chemotherapy. In two years of smoking it, he never had an adverse or untoward reaction. Marihuana was the least dangerous drug my husband received during the nine years he was treated for cancer.

During this period (1977–1979) Harris and I learned that many other cancer patients were smoking marihuana for the same purpose. Most of them had learned about it from their doctors, who could only offer hints and suggestions and rarely discussed the subject openly and thoroughly. They could not legally prescribe the drug to them or supervise their use of it, yet they could prescribe highly toxic chemotherapeutic drugs, dangerously addictive narcotics, and radiation treatments. I remember thinking how crazy it was.

Since Harris's death in 1979, I have had time to reflect on the meanness of a law that deprived him of his legal right to obtain the one drug that actually relieved his nausea and vomiting. I become upset, then enraged when I realize that other cancer patients are being denied such relief. I think about older people who might not know where to find marihuana or might be too frightened to smoke an illegal drug without close medical supervision. And I think about children and teenagers whose parents must face an agonizing choice between breaking the law and watching as their child suffers.

A final testimony to the powers of cannabis as an antiemetic, from Stephen Jay Gould, Alexander Professor of Geology at Harvard University and the author of many highly regarded books and essays on biological evolution:

> I am a member of a very small, very fortunate, and very select group—the first survivors of the previously incurable cancer, abdominal mesothelioma. Our treatment involved a carefully balanced mixture of all three standard modalities—surgery, radiation, and chemotherapy. Not pleasant, to be sure, but consider the alternative.
>
> Any cancer survivor of such intensive treatment—indeed, anyone who has endured aggressive medical battles against any disease—knows firsthand the enormous importance of the "psychological factor." Now I am an old-fashioned rationalist of the most unreconstructed sort. I brook no mysticism, no romantic Southern California nonsense about the power of mind and spirit. I assume that positive attitudes and optimism have salutary effects

because mental states can feed back upon the body through the immune system. In any case, I think that everyone would grant an important role to the maintenance of spirit through adversity; when the mind gives up, the body too often follows. (And if cure is not the ultimate outcome, quality of remaining life becomes, if anything, even more important.)

Nothing is more discouraging, more destructive of the possibility of such a positive attitude—and I do speak from personal experience here—than the serious side effects induced by so many treatments. Radiation and chemotherapy are often accompanied by long periods of intense and uncontrollable nausea. The mind begins to associate the agent of potential cure with the very worst aspect of the disease—for the pain and suffering of the side effects is often worse than the distress induced by the tumor itself. Once this happens, the possibility for an essential psychological boost and comfort may disappear—for the treatment seems worse than the disease itself. In other words, I am trying to say that the control of severe and long-lasting side effects in cancer treatment is not merely a question of comfort (though Lord only knows that comfort to the suffering is enough of a rationale), but an absolutely essential ingredient in the possibility of cure.

I had surgery, followed by a month of radiation, chemotherapy, more surgery, and a subsequent year of additional chemotherapy. I found that I could control the less severe nausea of radiation by conventional medicines. But when I started intravenous chemotherapy (Adriamycin®), absolutely nothing in the available arsenal of antiemetics worked at all. I was miserable and came to dread the frequent treatments with an almost perverse intensity.

I had heard that marihuana often worked well against nausea. I was reluctant to try it because I have never smoked any substance habitually (and didn't even know how to inhale). Moreover, I had tried marihuana twice (in the usual context of growing up in the sixties) and had hated it. (I am something of a Puritan on the subject of substances that, in any way, dull or alter mental states—for I value my rational mind with an academician's overweening arrogance. I do not drink alcohol at all, and have never used drugs in any "recreational" sense.) But anything to avoid nausea and the perverse wish it induces for an end of treatment. The rest of the story is short and sweet. Marihuana worked like a charm. I disliked the "side effect" of mental blurring (the "main effect" for recreational users), but the sheer bliss of not experiencing nausea—and then not having to fear it for all the days intervening between treatments—was the greatest boost I received in all my year of treatment, and surely had a most important effect upon my eventual cure. It is beyond my comprehension—and I fancy I am able to comprehend a lot, including much nonsense—that any humane person would withhold such a beneficial substance from people in such great need simply because others use it for different purposes.

Since 1985 oncologists have been legally permitted to administer synthetic THC orally in capsule form (Marinol®), and almost 100,000 doses were prescribed in 1989. But inhaled cannabis may be preferable for several reasons. Oral THC is erratically and slowly absorbed into the bloodstream. Furthermore, a patient who is severely nauseated and constantly vomiting may find it almost impossible to keep the capsule down. In 1979, Alfred Chang of the National Cancer Institute studied fifteen patients with bone cancer, comparing the antiemetic effects of oral and smoked delta-9-THC with corresponding placebos.[2] The patients served as their own controls. THC was clearly effective in reducing nausea and vomiting. Seventy-two percent of patients were nauseated and vomiting while taking a placebo. When the concentration of THC in their blood was low, 44 percent suffered from nausea and vomiting; at moderate concentrations, only 21 percent were nauseated and vomited; at fairly high concentrations just 6 percent did. Thus the effectiveness of THC depended on how

2. The THC was suspended in sesame oil and placed in gelatin capsules; seemingly identical placebo capsules contained only sesame oil. The placebo cigarettes contained marihuana from which the cannabinoids had been extracted; the active cigarettes were prepared from these placebo cigarettes by injecting THC through a needle.

much was absorbed into the bloodstream, and the investigators were able to show that smoked THC was absorbed more reliably.[3]

Most patients prefer smoked marihuana to oral THC, which makes them anxious and uncomfortable. One reason is the difficulty of titrating the dose of oral THC to control the amount that reaches the blood and brain. Another possibility, suggested by a group of Peruvian researchers, is that cannabidiol, one of the many substances in marihuana smoke, reduces anxiety provoked by delta-9-THC.[4] Thus, smoked marihuana may be both more effective and more comfortable to use than oral THC. We have already noted that patients in the state programs of the early 1980s almost universally preferred it.

In the spring of 1990 two investigators randomly selected more than two thousand members of the American Society of Clinical Oncology (one-third of the membership) and mailed them an anonymous questionnaire to learn their views on the use of cannabis in cancer chemotherapy. Almost half of the recipients responded. Although the investigators acknowledge that this group was self-selected and that there might be a response bias, their results provide a rough estimate of the views of specialists on the use of Marinol and smoked marihuana.

Only 43 percent said the available legal antiemetic drugs (including oral synthetic THC) provided adequate relief to all or most of their patients, and less than 46 percent said side effects of these drugs were a serious problem for only a few. Forty-four percent had recommended the illegal use of marihuana to at least one patient, and half would prescribe it to some patients if it were legal. On average, they considered smoked marihuana more effective than oral synthetic THC and roughly as safe.[5]

3. A. E. Chang et al., "Delta-9-tetrahydrocannabinol as an Antiemetic in Cancer Patients Receiving High-dose Methotrexate: A Prospective, Randomized Evaluation," *Annals of Internal Medicine* 91 (1979): 819–824.

4. A. W. Zuardi, I. Shirakawa, E. Finkelbarb, and I. G. Karniol, "Action of Cannabidiol on the Anxiety and Other Effects Produced by Delta-9-THC in Normal Subjects," *Psychopharmacology* 76 (1976): 245–250.

5. R. Doblin and M. A. R. Kleiman, "Marihuana as Anti-emetic Medicine: A Survey of Oncologists' Attitudes and Experiences," *Journal of Clinical Oncology* 9 (1991): 1275–1280.

One unfortunate effect of marihuana's illegality is that chemotherapy patients often have to learn how to use it on their own. It is not as simple as taking a pill; it may require some preparation and instruction, both to achieve the desired effect and to avoid undesired effects. Even oncologists who feel comfortable in recommending marihuana are usually ignorant about this. Patients may experience anxiety or even some degree of paranoia, especially if they do not know what to expect and how to titrate the dose. The psychoactive effects should be carefully explained so that patients will not be taken by surprise. Many will also require some explanation of the mechanics of smoking. Once marihuana becomes an accepted medical treatment for nausea and vomiting, few patients will experience difficulty or discomfort in using it.

GLAUCOMA

Glaucoma is a disorder that results from an imbalance of pressure within the eye. The eyeball must be almost perfectly spherical to focus light accurately on the retina. Its shape is maintained by the pressure of an internal fluid, the aqueous humor. If the eye produces too much of this fluid or if the channels through which the fluid flows out are blocked, the increasing pressure may damage the optic nerve, which carries impulses from the eye to the brain. Glaucoma afflicts 1.5 percent of the population at age fifty and about 5 percent at age seventy. Except for degeneration of the retina in old age, it is the leading cause of blindness in the United States, accounting for 10 percent of adult-onset cases. Most glaucoma is of the open-angle or chronic simple type, in which the channels narrow gradually and the pressure within rises slowly. The resulting loss of peripheral vision may go unnoticed until the disease is well advanced. Early detection and careful monitoring and control of intraocular pressure are necessary to avoid irreversible damage.

Today glaucoma is treated chiefly with eyedrops containing beta-blockers, which inhibit the activity of epinephrine (adrenaline). They are highly effective but may have serious side effects; they may induce depression, aggravate asthma, slow the heart rate, and increase the risk of heart failure. Paradoxically, epinephrine-like eyedrops can also be effective in treating glaucoma, but they may irritate the white of the eye and aggravate hypertension and heart disease. Miotics (drugs that contract the pupil), such as pilocarpine, are also prescribed for glaucoma, although less often now than in the past. They are generally safe for the heart, respiratory, and digestive system but can cause blurred vision, impaired night vision, and cataracts. Patients may also be given pills containing a carbonic anhydrase inhibitor, which reduces the production of aqueous humor. Carbonic anhydrase inhibitors may cause loss of appetite, nausea, diarrhea, headaches, numbness and tingling, depression and fatigue, kidney stones, and, rarely, a fatal blood disorder. Fifty percent of glaucoma patients cannot tolerate the side effects of these drugs.

The discovery that marihuana reduces intraocular pressure occurred accidentally during an experiment at the University of California at Los Angeles designed to determine whether, as the Los Angeles Police Department believed, cannabis dilated the pupils; the police claimed that this supposed dilation (along with, among another things, white lips and a green-coated tongue) was a sign of marihuana intoxication and therefore good grounds for arresting and searching a citizen. The subjects of the experiment were normal volunteers smoking government-grown marihuana. Their eyes were photographed as they smoked, and the pupils were found to be slightly constricted rather than dilated. An ophthalmological examination showed that cannabis also reduced tearing (users have often claimed that they can comfortably chop onions while high) and intraocular pressure. Further experiments indicated a similar effect in patients with glaucoma.[6] Marihuana reduced intraocular pressure for an average of four to five hours, with "no indications of any deleterious effects . . . on visual function or ocular structure."[7] Under

6. R. S. Hepler and I. M. Frank, "Marihuana Smoking and Intraocular Pressure," *JAMA* 217 (1971): 1392.
    7. Ibid.

its influence the pupils responded normally to light; visual acuity, refraction, peripheral visual fields, binocular vision, and color vision were not affected. The researchers concluded that marihuana may be more useful than conventional medications and probably works by a different mechanism. This conclusion has been confirmed by further human experiments and animal studies.

The effect on intraocular pressure occurs when marihuana is smoked or THC is taken orally. In one study, nineteen patients smoked marihuana for thirty-five days and another twenty-nine patients smoked it for ninety-four days without developing tolerance to the effect on intraocular pressure or any deterioration of vision.[8] Several animal studies have established that cannabis is also active when applied topically (that is, as an eyedrop). This is important, because topical application has fewer psychological effects and is more acceptable to ophthalmologists. Unfortunately, cannabis preparations suitable for topical application in human beings have not yet been developed.

In the phase known as end-stage glaucoma, the patient has already lost a substantial degree of vision, the condition is worsening, standard drugs are no longer effective, and blindness is imminent. The writer of the following account, Robert Randall, had reached that stage when he began to smoke marihuana regularly. He had used all the available glaucoma drugs at the highest permitted doses, and his intraocular pressure remained dangerously high. If nothing further had been done, he would have gone blind.

I smoked my first marihuana cigarette the day Richard Nixon was elected President. Jerry Ford was President when I smoked my first legal "research" joint. Jimmy Carter was elected days before I walked out of a Washington, D.C., hospital carrying the nation's first modern prescription for medical marihuana. I

8. R. S. Hepler, I. M. Frank, and R. Petrus, "Ocular Effects of Marihuana Smoking," in *The Pharmacology of Marihuana*, ed. M. C. Braude and S. Szara, 2 vols. (New York: Raven, 1976), 2:815–824.

legally toked through the Reagan years, unscathed by the mindless War on Drugs. George Bush is President now. I still legally smoke medicinal marihuana and, as a result, still enjoy my sight.

My stepping stones to the wacky weed were alcohol and tobacco. I began smoking tobacco because I wanted to smoke pot and needed practice inhaling. A purely economic decision; tobacco then cost two cents a cigarette. Marihuana, by comparison, was obscenely expensive—fifteen to twenty dollars an ounce for the really good stuff. I was hooked on sweet nicotine after my first cigarette—an attraction I have yet to resolve.

Marihuana, of course, was profoundly different. It was far safer, nonaddictive, and illegal. Unlike many first time tokers, I got blitzed. When I closed my eyes I saw glossy Kodachrome snaps—mental ViewMaster slides—of good friends looking very happy indeed. In another culture this might be interpreted as the weed's way of saying I needed the good it could afford. I enjoyed marihuana very much. It was fun.

My life underwent subtle, pervasive changes. First, an alteration in sensory inputs. Agonizingly loud, over-bright booze binges involving herds of highly intoxicated people were replaced by quiet evenings sitting in semi-darkness within a small circle of close confidants—fellow criminals against Empire all—listening to hard rock played low so as not to arouse suspicion, a towel stuffed under the door to avoid apprehension.

I cruised through college on clouds of cannabis, completed my undergraduate work early and started my master's. No problems in the academy. Most of my friends smoked. I enjoyed smoking marihuana in groups or alone, learned to revel in the suddenly plastic character of thought. The marihuana-induced jump from hyper-linear sequencing to the universe of randomly interconnected thoughts and obtuse associations delighted me. McLuhan rendered comprehensible. Finally, when I smoked marihuana I saw more clearly. I'm not talking enlightenment. I'm talking sight. Seeing. Since my mid-teens my evenings had been haunted by minor visual problems—transient tricolored halos. On some evenings I would go white-blind, my vision snared in an impenetrable swirl of absolute illumination—the white void.

I knew these problems were minor because when I noted them to my physicians they told me if I was older it might be serious. But, since I was too young for it to be serious, it must be "eye strain." All that diligent study. If they weren't worried, why should I be? Particularly since marihuana relaxed my "eye strain." Nothing special in that. Marihuana relaxes nearly everything: mind, body, soul. That chronic kink in the neck. So why not eye strain? Without marihuana to ease my "eye strain" I probably could not have completed my master's.

Following graduation in 1971, I moved to Washington to write stirring speeches for powerful people and ended up driving a cab. I loved driving a cab. Most instructive. No boss. You set your own hours. I'd also stopped smoking marihuana. Being in a new city, surrounded by new people, I had few friends and no access—no dealer.

One evening in the summer of 1972, I closed my left eye and discovered I could not read with my right eye. Instead of clearly formed letters I saw a jumble of black ink splashed on a white page. No matter how close I drew the text, it remained indecipherable, incoherent, alien. Someone gave me the name of a good ophthalmologist. I saw him the following afternoon. I was twenty-four.

Benjamin Fine, M.D., one of the nation's leading ocular pathologists, performed a number of tests. I told him of my halos and white-blindness. His assistant took me through my first visual field examination. Eventually, the doctor called me to his inner office. There was grimness in his manner. Clearly, not good news.

Said Dr. Fine, "Son, you have a very serious condition called glaucoma. You have already suffered a lot of visual damage and . . ."

"How long?"

Thrown by my directness, he responded in kind: "At best

you've got three, maybe five years of remaining sight. You've lost most of the vision in both eyes. Your right eye has no central vision—no reading vision—none. In your left eye you only have a small island of healthy tissue. That's why you can read. Your pressure in both eyes is over forty. It should be under twenty. You are in very, very serious trouble. You are going to go blind."

Surgery was risky, especially in someone with my advanced level of damage. There was a good chance surgery would annihilate the small fragments of healthy optic tissue which remained.

"I'm sorry, son. We'll do the best we can, but there's not a lot we can do. You are going to go blind." He looked worn out. Doctor Fine put pilocarpine in my eyes, gripped me by the shoulders, asked if I was all right, gave me a pat on the back, and sent me out the door with those most fateful words: "Just live life like you always have . . ." Patients know the end to this dreaded sentence, "because you won't have it for long."

Generally unfazed by this most pessimistic meeting on the future of my life I wandered downstairs, got in my cab, and realized I could not see beyond the dashboard. Pilocarpine, a miotic, induces intense nearsightedness. I drove through D.C. rush-hour traffic guided by memory and the glare of sunlight off the cars in front of me.

I ignored this gaping invitation to debilitating depression. I could still see, still read, still softly fondle all nature's hues and tones. Until, of course, I put in my newly prescribed Pilo [pilocarpine], which quickly reduced my sight to remnants of ill-defined shape. My introduction to the wonderfully twisted world of glaucoma pharmacology.

Medically seeking to preserve sight by employing drugs which induce functional blindness results in what physicians disdainfully call "patient noncompliance." This means if I really wanted to see a movie I'd stop taking Pilo, shrug off my pharmaceutically induced myopia and enjoy the film. You might lose some sight, but at least you could see the flick.

Glaucoma and its therapies introduced me to much larger,

more disruptive realities. Pilo and driving don't mix. Within a week of diagnosis, I was out of my cab and out of work. Deemed "disabled," I landed on welfare, an unexpected ward of the state. This really was getting serious.

Within weeks of diagnosis, my prescription for Pilo doubled, redoubled, tripled, quadrupled. Within months, epinephrine was added. Epi caused my heart to race, opened my pupils wide, and let in such a flood of photons I felt I was drowning in light. Then came Diamox [a carbonic anhydrase inhibitor], a pill, a diuretic. Crushing fatigue. The taste of everything changed. Finally, in desperation, phospholine iodide, an eyedrop developed from a World War II nerve gas, was added to the mix. This battering pharmaceutical assault left me blurry-eyed, dysfunctionally myopic, photophobic, extremely tired, with a chronic backache— calcification of my kidneys. Objective medical control over elevated intraocular pressures (IOP), however, remained elusive. My rapidly escalating intake of toxic prescriptions was outraced by the dynamic character of my glaucoma. Each visual field shrank.

Despite my use of every pharmaceutical agent in the inventory, my evenings were routinely visited by tricolored halos— a signature of ocular pressures over 35 mm Hg [millimeters of mercury]. On some nights the halos were muted. On other evenings they appeared as hard crystal rings emanating from every source of light. And then there were nights, not so rare, of white-blindness—the world rendered invisible by its brilliance. Clinical translation: ocular tension in excess of 40 mm Hg. To summarize, things were not going very well.

Then someone gave me a couple of joints. Sweet weed! That night I made and ate dinner, watched television. My tricolored halos arrived, which made watching TV less interesting. So I put on some good music, dimmed offending lights, and got into some serious toking. I happened to look out my window at a distant street lamp and noticed what was not there. No halos. That's when I had the full blown, omni-dimensional technicolor cartoon light-bulb experience. In a transcendent instant the spheres spoke! So simple. Old messages—new context. You smoke pot, your eye strain goes away. Ganja is good for you.

Sure was fun, but in the medicated haze of the next miotic morning I chided my raging rapture and began a baseline reality check. My well-educated, acutely dispassionate intellect was not kind. "Let us," my left sphere said, "be analytical." Brace yourself—the facts are not pretty. This poor, super-stressed soul, unwilling to accept the cumulative horror of what has become "real life," gets his hands on some really good pot. He smokes a couple of joints and gets a bit dopey. OK, certifiably Fruit Loops. In despair and desperation, he imagines marihuana is going to "save his sight."

Are we crazy? The answer is obvious, right? Given these facts, who would not want to believe something mystical, magical, mysterious, and forbidden is going to rescue them from the pit of eternal darkness? The idea that a legally prohibited, medically unavailable weed—a plant smoked for sheer delight, for fun—is going to "save your sight" is madcap and reckless; as farfetched, improbable, and pathetic a notion as someone insane could imagine. So began six months of cynical observation. Six months of simple trial and error. At the end, the conclusion was unavoidable. Without marihuana there were halos and white-blind nights. When I smoked marihuana there were no halos. Is a pattern emerging? You bet. If I watched very closely I could actually observe the halos depart. The cumulative evidence of a reproducible benefit was inescapable.

So, I accept that an illegal, medically prohibited weed may help me not go blind. What now? Do I rush to introduce nice, middle-aged, middle-of-the-road, prestigious ocular pathologist and genuinely swell fellow, Dr. Ben Fine, to my pot-driven revelation, which is, of course, of potential benefit to millions of similarly afflicted humans? Yeah, right! No way! He's a good doctor. I like him. He's honest. But he would not appreciate my news. There are medical questions. And, of course, legal concerns. Like malpractice or worse. If Dr. Fine knows but does not tell the police, does he become my criminal accomplice? A co-conspirator? "Pot Doc arrested!" His career in ruins.

If not my trusted doctor, then whom? I could tell the drug bureaucrats? Sure! "Marihuana Can Be Good For You!" This is just the sort of good news rabid antidrug zealots are longing to hear. In this very unsubtle way, fear—prohibition-induced fear—pervades any dialogue on marihuana's medical use, separating patients from physicians, from other patients, from government. You are isolated. In the best of times, under the best of circumstances, this is not something to be wished for. When you are young and going blind, the inability to share such vital information with the physician treating you or with others who might be helped becomes downright scary. It became a time of simple goals. Keep smoking, keep your mouth shut, and stay sighted. Seeing is real. Everything else is politics.

Doctor Fine, though mystified by the sudden change in my condition, was greatly pleased by the results. My ever-eroding visual fields stabilized. My slide into darkness slowed, then halted. As my glaucoma came under medical management, other aspects of life began to right themselves. I escaped welfare and took a part-time teaching job at a local college.

Discounting unsavory encounters with underworld characters, illegal marihuana is frightfully expensive, absolutely unregulated, and not always available. To cope with the uncertainty of adequate supply I did what many patients still do. I grew some pot.

In 1974 I tried cultivating cannabis indoors, only to watch as devouring squadrons of spider mites euphorically consumed my entire crop. The next spring two small marihuana plants— the product of seeds unintentionally dropped the year before— sprouted through the boards of my sun deck. We re-potted the seeds, planted a few more, then watched nature do the rest. By midsummer we were blessed by beautiful six-foot pot plants. Things were going swell. My vision was stable. I was employed. I'd rediscovered loose change. Alice had come to live with me. Swell. These were the last quiet days of my life.

While we were vacationing in Indiana, the local vice cops raided my house and seized my six-foot marihuana plants. I returned to find a warrant on the kitchen table with a note scribbled on the back requesting that I surrender myself for arrest. I could not know at the time, but being arrested was about the best thing that could have happened to me. Being arrested "saved my sight."

When I told my attorneys I was smoking marihuana to treat my glaucoma, they thought it was hysterical. When they realized I was not joking, they stopped laughing only long enough to tell me to prove it. I spoke with Keith Stroup, head of the National Organization for the Reform of Marihuana Laws. Keith didn't laugh. Instead, he carefully explained that I didn't have a prayer. But he gave me a few phone numbers and suggested I phone around. So I phoned around the federal bureaucracy. Needless to say, I was startled when at least three bureaucrats point-blank told me, "Oh, we know marihuana helps glaucoma. We have lots of data which shows . . ." They knew! They knew and hadn't bothered to tell me. They knew, but did not want anyone else to know. Remember, this is 1975, not yesterday.

Given a choice between administering a reckless, well-established absolute and catholic prohibition or honestly meeting the urgent medical needs of desperately ill citizens, the drug bureaucrats had, of course, chosen deceit to maintain their institutionally treasured fraud. This is why bureaucrats the world 'round are so beloved by the citizens they serve.

Proving that marihuana lowers intraocular pressures is not difficult. The government, my government, was fully aware of marihuana's beneficial effects on glaucoma by early 1971. Marihuana is a political issue, not a mere medical matter. Besides, you cannot make a profit growing medicinal weeds. The medical mandarins occupying the National Eye Institute did not wish to get involved. They, too, were afraid. It might hurt funding. When I requested help, NEI refused to conduct any experiments with marihuana because I might want to use the data in court.

The nation's leading ocular specialists were politically correct and very anti-marihuana. Besides, the doctors said thoughtfully, you could never use marihuana. Marihuana causes people to "get high." And we all know just how life-threatening euphoria can be.

Eventually I underwent two highly controlled medical experiments. The first, conducted at the Jules Stein Eye Institute, UCLA, required my incarceration in a mental ward for thirteen days of round-the-clock observation. I arrived in the middle of an ongoing research project involving six "routine" research subjects who were being tested on pure synthetic THC—a man-made copy of marihuana's most mind-altering chemical. The UCLA researchers did more than simply confirm that marihuana lowered my ocular tension. They discovered that my disease could not be controlled using conventional glaucoma medicines. Left on these drugs I would go blind, just as Dr. Fine predicted. I was also tested on synthetic THC [Marinol]. What a lousy, marginal drug! The "high" is anxiety-provoking. The therapeutic effects, if any, are minimal, transient, unpredictable. But THC comes in a pill. The bureaucrats, the research scientists and doctors can relate to pills. Besides, we all know you shouldn't smoke. In the end, UCLA determined marihuana was not merely beneficial; it was critical to the medical maintenance of my vision.

OK. It's proved. Let's go to court. I was ready, but my anxious attorneys conspired with an even more anxiety-ridden Dr. Fine to compel me into a second, confirmatory evaluation. On the Ides of March, 1976, a second, much less fun experiment was undertaken at the Wilmer Eye Institute, Johns Hopkins University, where I was institutionalized for six of the most miserable days of my existence. The Wilmer physicians were under strict instructions from Dr. Fine to find a conventional solution. He didn't want to testify in court. So they threw every glaucoma drug in the book at my condition. I wandered into the medical library, where I became alarmed by the cumulative adverse effects commonplace among chronic users of glaucoma medicines. A brief list would include cataracts, kidney stones, gastric ulcers, skin rashes, drug fevers, mental confusion, abrupt mood swings, hypertension, renal, respiratory, or cardiac failure, death. The Wilmer Eye Institute physicians, despite their seemingly perverse glee in exposing me to highly toxic medicines, could not conduct an evaluation of marihuana. No government clearance. No grant. In the midst of this meanness a most curious thing happened. I got to know my roomie, a fifty-three-year-old West Virginia factory worker named Vince. We had just met, barely exchanged hellos, when Vince asked, "You tried any good marihuana?" Blown away?! You bet. Seems ole Vince had taken a break with a couple of his night shift buddies and smoked weed for the first time in his life. Bingo! Vince noticed his halos went away. "If I could get my hands on enough marihuana, I sure as hell wouldn't be in here," Vince convincingly said. Two days later I watched the guys in white wheel Vince into cryosurgery, a ghastly, painful procedure which freezes, kills, a part of the eye in an effort to reduce ocular pressure. That night Vince groaned in agony; his toes curled in torment. After leaving Wilmer I followed Vince's progress for quite some time. The mutilating surgery had not helped him. Eventually, unable to "get enough marihuana," Vince went blind.

I had been in glaucoma therapy for nearly four years, and Vince was the first glaucoma patient I'd ever met. And Vince knew! How many others knew? At the conclusion of their pharmaceutical torment, the Wilmer doctors grudgingly conceded failure. UCLA's evaluation was correct: in the absence of marihuana my ocular tension was beyond medical control. Ignoring the UCLA data on marihuana, the Wilmer surgeons recommended immediate surgical intervention.

What a surprise! Without marihuana I would go blind. Everyone agreed on that. The Wilmer physicians, in their zeal to evade this fact, had recommended surgical procedures Dr. Fine knew would result in blindness. He finally agreed to testify in my defense. He took the very highest ground; given the facts, it would be medically unethical to withhold marihuana. The rest, as they say, is history. Briefly summarized:

- In May 1976, I petitioned federal drug agencies for immediate access to government supplies of marihuana.
- In July, at my trial, we raised the untried legal defense of "medical necessity." Essentially, a simple argument that any sane soul who is going blind would break the law to save his sight.
- In November 1976, the bureaucrats cracked. They delivered a tin of three hundred pre-rolled marihuana cigarettes to my new doctor, John Merritt at Howard University. In this way I became the first American to gain legal, medically supervised access to marihuana.
- In the same month, the D.C. Superior Court ruled my use of marihuana was not criminal, but an act of "medical necessity." It was the first successful articulation of the "medical necessity" defense in the history of English Common Law.

My first year of smoking was not tranquil. In fact, it turned into a running battle. I'd speak out. The bureaucrats would try to clamp down. Very unpleasant. Increasing news coverage unhinged the bureaucrats. Other patients were expecting help. By early 1978, the feds hit the wall, bit the bullet and cut off my legal line of supply. I countered by suing. Twenty-four hours after the suit was filed, we arrived at an out-of-court settlement which is still in effect. This settlement assures me of medically appropriate (non-research) access to marihuana to meet my legitimate therapeutic needs.

Elvy Musikka is a woman in her mid-forties who lives in Hollywood, Florida. This is her story:

In late February 1975 I went to see Dr. Rosenfeld, a general practitioner in the Ft. Lauderdale area. He concluded a very thorough examination and said my eyes had been stricken with glaucoma. My [intraocular fluid] pressures were in the high 40s [pressure in the low teens is normal], and Dr. Rosenfeld insisted I see an ophthalmologist immediately. His suspicions were confirmed and I was started on pilocarpine eyedrops.

By the spring of 1976 the pilocarpine itself was becoming a problem. I began seeing circles but assumed they were a symptom of the glaucoma. Wearing contact lenses was uncomfortable and my pressures were going up. A new doctor suggested I consider marihuana because it was likely that otherwise I would go blind. He told me this as a friend, not a doctor; it was then that I began to realize that sometimes doctors have to choose between Hippocratic oaths and hypocritical laws. I was most fortunate this man had a heart.

Blindness was not new to me. I was born blind, with congenital cataracts, and had my first eye surgery at five. Surgery then was very different from the laser surgery of today, and I was left with a lot of scar tissue. I wore very thick glasses until fourteen or so, when I had surgery on my left eye. Something went wrong and I lost most of my sight in that eye. But with 20/200 vision in the right eye and the help of contact lenses, I had gotten along quite well, until this most recent finding.

I was uncomfortable with the thought of taking marihuana, a drug I had been misinformed to believe was as dangerous and addictive as heroin. Because of my anxiety, the first time I used it I became sick to my stomach. I find that particularly amusing now, as I have discovered that it is very effective in preventing and alleviating nausea. I have also discovered that, like myself at first, some people feel paranoid after using marihuana, but now I wonder whether this is an effect of the plant itself or due to longstanding myths about its dangerousness. I don't get paranoid using it any more—maybe that is a clue?

That summer I discovered something curious. One day I visited the doctor scared to death because my friend Jerry and I had spent an awful lot of the night before drinking champagne. I presumed it would have increased my pressures, and was very surprised to find that they were 12 and 13. My doctor explained that downers such as alcohol, marihuana, and Demerol bring pressures down. He felt the safest of the three was marihuana.

I was having a terrible time smoking it, so my doctor and I decided it would be best for me to take it in brownies instead. He warned I would need a bit more than smoking. He gave me a recipe that called for an ounce of marihuana to yield a batch of twenty-four brownies—a twelve-day supply.

I didn't know where to go for marihuana and didn't always have access to it. Once my pressures were so high my doctor obtained some for me. It was handled through his secretary. Oh, that poor woman! How she shook! Her hands were ice cold when she handed me the bag. I thanked God for these compassionate people. I knew the street value was thirty to forty dollars an ounce but she only took fifteen dollars. That couldn't continue, of course, and I sought to obtain marihuana legally.

I couldn't find enough, and had to keep using pilocarpine. When it started making me see circles again, my doctor was out of town, and I went to a new clinic. When the attending physician there realized that I was using marihuana to treat my glaucoma, he looked very disgusted. He threw two prescriptions at me and sent me home without instructions and warnings. Those two drugs were the most horrible I have ever come across in my life. Diamox took all the potassium out of my body and I was completely apathetic. My children had to care for themselves because when I came home I could only go to bed. At the time I did not have the money to buy the second prescription, phospholine iodide, which I eventually tried and found unbearably painful.

I called my hometown newspaper and told a reporter about my use of marihuana in a telephone interview. I spoke without giving my name or picture, because I feared losing my job and custody of my children. But a lot of people recognized the story as mine and came forward, confessing that they were regular marihuana smokers and would help me get marihuana when possible. You can imagine my shock! Some of these people were co-workers, others respected members of the community. None of them—not a one—was a bum as I had been led to think of every marihuana smoker.

In January 1977 my doctor sent me to a research center at the University of Miami. He thought they might help me obtain marihuana legally. But the very dedicated scientists at the center didn't want to hear the "m" word. Instead, I spent one of the most grueling days of my life. When I arrived my pressures were in the high 50s in the right eye and high 40s in the left. They gave me everything they could think of. Drops didn't help much, nor did using a little pump to flush the eye. I also had to drink a big glass of a sickeningly sweet liquid, which didn't help either. At the day's end my pressures had barely lowered to the 40s, so I was scheduled for emergency surgery.

At home that night I used a remaining bit of marihuana to bake some brownies, and ate two every twelve hours. The doctors were shocked when they checked my pressures as I arrived for surgery the next Monday morning—perfectly normal at 14 and 16! Regardless, they readied me for surgery, even though it had at best a 30 percent chance of helping me! The following morning they performed an operation on my tear ducts which turned out to be of no value. Because of it I now have to wear the big magnifying glasses that I had managed to avoid since childhood. After this procedure I had less sight, more scar tissue, and higher pressures, and I was unable to return to work.

I now faced not only glaucoma but depression and poverty. It would be at least nine months before Social Security could issue a disability check. I was humiliated using food stamps but glad they were available. I developed insomnia. Marihuana was harder to find now that I had no money to buy it. Sometimes compassionate people gave me some and my insomnia disappeared. It was certainly the best antidepressant I have ever come across.

By 1980 I had little money and marihuana had gone up in price, so I started growing my own plants. I used the finest seeds, which produced small plants, hard to detect but productive. I only required three or four joints a day. My pressures became so close to normal that my doctors decided a corneal transplant was safe. It worked! I never have had such beautiful eyesight—it was so wonderful! I was so happy, until neighbors jumped the fence around my yard and stole my marihuana plants.

My pressures went sky high, and I escaped into alcohol quite a bit of the time. When I started having slight blackouts I realized alcohol was not the answer. So reluctantly and fearfully I went through surgery again. This time I hemorrhaged and before I knew it, my right eye was blind. Since I had only 20/400 vision in my left eye, you could have lit up my bedroom with bright lights as I slept and I wouldn't have awakened. I was very depressed. Most painful were the happy dreams in which I was seeing out of both eyes and being the person I used to be. Then I would wake up to find myself without the right eye.

I needed money and had an extra room in my house, so I put an ad in the paper and acquired a boarder. He assured me he was not taking illegal drugs and would not tell anyone I was growing marihuana. But soon his erratic behavior convinced me there was a problem, and sure enough, I found cocaine under the bathroom sink. At first he denied using drugs, but a few days later he admitted it. He said he needed cocaine because in his job as a car salesman he was expected to work seven days a week, ten hours a day. I told him that I didn't care about his reasons; he would have to move. He agreed that he would, but as the time grew closer he became reluctant. We argued, and he turned me in to the police.

I was arrested on the night of March 4, 1988, and it changed my life forever. I notified the media, and this time my hometown paper photographed me and wrote a full follow-up story. I was contacted by people who had obtained marihuana legally, and my doctor and his secretary spent at least fifty hours on paperwork to be submitted to the DEA, FDA, and NIDA in an effort to secure legal marihuana. I did a lot of radio shows, and it was always heartbreaking because almost always, there was someone who had lost their sight unnecessarily. There were also genuinely concerned citizens who worried about my being addicted to a horrible drug and who sincerely wished that there was another answer for me. Of course, they hadn't been me and they hadn't been on it for twelve years, so they didn't realize that there were no side effects for me to fear. I began to hear from people all over the country, even some from Canada. It was amazing; many were glaucoma patients who had maintained their sight for twenty and twenty-five years with marihuana and are still illegally maintaining it today. I envied them for standing up for their health, for knowing what they were doing and taking care of themselves.

But that was no help to me now. I was facing felony charges. In Florida, possession of anything over twenty grams is a felony, and they confiscated an ounce and a half from a plant I had just harvested the previous Monday.

My trial began and ended August 15, 1988. I knew one thing: if I was going to court, so was this unjust law. I was not afraid. I felt that God and his angels were with me. I was not mistaken—the only person they could find to testify against me was the arresting officer, and I wouldn't say he was against me. Glaucoma patients testified on my behalf, and my doctor proclaimed marihuana the only agent that ever provided reliable relief for me. I was asked if I had smoked marihuana since my arrest and I answered yes. "Did you smoke marihuana today?" "Of course," I replied. The judge listened carefully and decided that for me not to have tried to preserve whatever sight I had left would have been total insanity. He said that I had no intent of criminal activity, and I was acquitted. I had applied for a Compassionate IND in March 1988 and was granted legal use of marihuana provided by the government beginning October 21, 1988.

The sight in my right eye is coming back. I now have perceptions of light, colors, and shapes. In my left eye, which used to be 20/400 but is now 20/100, the optic nerve is very healthy and I have lost no peripheral vision. As a matter of fact it has improved. Miraculous—that's cannabis.

EPILEPSY

Epilepsy is a condition in which certain brain cells (the epileptic focus) become abnormally excitable and spontaneously discharge in an uncontrolled way, causing a seizure. In grand mal or generalized epilepsy, the abnormal cells are on both sides of the brain and the discharge produces convulsions (violent muscle spasms). In absence seizures, the generalized brain discharge causes a lapse of consciousness but not convulsions. Partial seizures result from abnormal discharge in an isolated area of the brain and may occur with or without a change in consciousness.

Partial seizures with a change in consciousness, known as complex partial seizures, are caused by damage to the temporal or frontal lobes of the cerebral cortex. They were formerly known as psychomotor seizures, because the symptoms also include motor activity (grimacing and repetitive mouth or hand movements are especially common). When overexcitation is confined to a very small area, the patient with epilepsy may have a strange sensation of déja vu, vertigo, fear, or an odd smell without a source. This experience, known as an aura, may or may not be followed by a full complex partial seizure.

Epilepsy is treated primarily with anticonvulsant drugs, but they help only about 75 percent of the time. Focal seizures and temporal lobe epilepsy in particular are difficult to treat with standard anticonvulsants.[9] Furthermore, anticonvulsant drugs have potentially serious side effects, including bone softening, pernicious anemia (reduced production of red blood cells), swelling of the gums, and emotional disturbances. Overdoses or idiosyncratic reactions may cause nystagmus (rapid uncontrollable eye movements), loss of motor coordination, coma, and even death.[10]

Although the anticonvulsant properties of cannabis have been known since ancient times and were explored in the nineteenth cen-

9. P. Robb, "Focal Epilepsy: The Problem, Prevalence, and Contributing Factors," *Advanced Neurology* 8 (1975): 11–22.

10. H. Kutt and S. Louis, "Untoward Effects of Anticonvulsants," *New England Journal of Medicine* 286 (1972): 1316–1317.

tury, this therapeutic use of the drug has been largely ignored in the past hundred years. A rare exception is a short paper by J. P. Davis and H. H. Ramsey published in 1949. They studied the effects of two tetrahydrocannabinol congeners on five institutionalized children with severe grand mal epilepsy that was inadequately controlled by the standard anticonvulsant drugs phenobarbital and phenytoin (Dilantin®). Three did no worse than before; the fourth became almost completely free of seizures and the fifth entirely so.[11]

The medical literature was again silent on this topic until 1975, when the following case of grand mal epilepsy was reported:

> A 24-year-old man has been seen in a neurology outpatient clinic for a period of eight years for control of his epileptic seizures. His history included febrile convulsions at three years of age and epileptic seizures since the age of 16. Since that age the patient has been taking diphenylhydantoin sodium (phenytoin), 100 mg. four times a day, and phenobarbital, 30 mg. four times a day. Control of seizures with this regimen was incomplete, and the patient complained of attacks about once every two months. From the age of 16 to 22, the incidence of seizures increased from one attack per month to one per week.
>
> At 22 years of age the patient began smoking marihuana (two to five joints per night) while continuing the prescribed anticonvulsant drug therapy. During this period, attacks did not occur as long as the patient continued to take the combination of all three drugs. The patient's condition could not be maintained on marihuana alone, because on two occasions he experienced an attack three to four days after running out of his prescribed medication.[12]

In a later study, sixteen patients with grand mal epilepsy who were not responding well to treatment were given 200 to 300 milligrams

11. J. P. Davis and H. H. Ramsey, "Antiepileptic Action of Marijuana-active Substances," *Federation Proceedings* 8 (1949): 284–285.
12. P. F. Consroe, G. C. Wood, and H. Buchsbaum, "Anticonvulsant Nature of Marihuana Smoking," *JAMA* 234 (1975): 306–307.

of cannabidiol or a placebo in addition to their antiepileptic drugs. After five months, three of the cannabidiol patients showed complete improvement, two exhibited partial improvement, and two showed minor improvement; one was unchanged. Mild sedation was the only side effect. Of the placebo patients, only one improved substantially and seven were unchanged. The researchers concluded that for some patients cannabidiol combined with standard antiepileptics may be useful in controlling seizures. Whether cannabidiol alone, in large doses, would be helpful is not known.[13]

Although the medical establishment continues to show little interest, more and more epilepsy sufferers are discovering the usefulness of cannabis. Carl Oglesby has a complex partial seizure disorder; the seizure arises in the temporal lobe and spreads, but remains relatively focal:

> In 1972, at the age of thirty-seven, I discovered that marihuana medicated a seizure that had plagued me since my teenage years and for which no legal medication seemed available. Shortly after that I became a daily user. Today, because I am uncomfortable with the legal risks of using marihuana, I am resolved to find a different way to deal with my problem.
>
> My seizure first appeared when I was fifteen or sixteen and has persisted to my current age of fifty-four at a rate varying from a half-dozen to two dozen episodes a day. Episodes vary in duration (from half a minute to a minute) and in intensity, but never in form. There are always two stages. The first is an onset or aura stage, and the second is defined by the facial spasm that forms the crux of the seizure.
>
> The first warning comes as a subtle yet ineffably corporeal sensation, an uh-oh feeling, distinctly unpleasant, of lightness and airiness, a kind of inner tickling with a throbbing, giddy quality. It is centered in my chest at first, but diffuses into my head within

13. J. M. Cunha, E. A. Carlini, A. E. Pereira, et al., "Chronic Administration of Cannabidiol to Healthy Volunteers and Epileptic Patients," *Pharmacology* 21 (1980): 175–185.

a few seconds and incorporates the entire background of mental activity. That is, I can still talk and sustain a line of thought, but it requires special effort because of an inclusive if private sense of alarm.

I am aware of some physical displays that I cannot control during the onset. My nostrils flare, my eyes dance and sparkle, my voice tightens and its pitch becomes erratic, my diaphragm contracts, my breathing becomes irregular, and I feel vaguely disoriented. It is as though my body becomes excited, almost pleasantly so, but without any social or mental correlative, context, or motive. Since the loss of physical control over oneself is always disconcerting, an experience that bears a certain gross resemblance to glee becomes a source of helplessness and dread.

The seizure proper emerges as a crescendo from the aura and is partly an intensification of the aura. Its dominant component, however, is a physically irresistible grin that takes over the entire right side of my face without affecting the left side at all. Everything else about the seizure, as far as I can tell, is bilateral: both eyes sparkle, both sides of my diaphragm contract, both nostrils flare. But this uniformly right-sided rictus is the ground zero of the seizure, the point and climax toward which the aura phase ascends. The aura stage is essentially private and easily concealed, but the rictus subjects me to social penalties. I can conceal it only by hiding my face or diverting attention from myself.

When the seizure first appeared, I could not understand or explain it and felt too ashamed to ask for help. My parents, unsophisticated people, reprimanded me for what my father called my "silly grin" (as in "get that silly grin off your face"). When I tried to explain it to my friends, they responded that I should laugh if I felt like laughing. I couldn't make them understand that I didn't feel like laughing—or that, perhaps, yes, I did, but the feeling came over me as though from elsewhere and had no connection with any thought or perception or ordinary motivation. I could not convey this sense of externality, of being seized by a motive beyond consciousness.

So I gave up, resolved to keep this shameful thing, my silly grin, as much to myself as possible, and developed a repertoire of concealments. I credit myself with not becoming reclusive. I debated in high school and college, took up work that kept me in constant contact with other people, and later, in my early thirties, played a leading role (as president of Students for a Democratic Society, SDS) in opposing the Vietnam War. I even performed on stage for several years in college and loved it, although I eventually had to concede that the seizure made acting impossible.

If a seizure threatened at an inopportune moment—which happened constantly—I had a variety of responses. If I was holding the floor, I would divert attention from myself somehow, often simply by asking someone a question. If necessary I would stage a little choking fit, pick up a glass of water, and use it as a prop to help conceal the rictus. In other settings I might conveniently discover a piece of apple stuck in an upper molar on the right side of my mouth. I let only my most intimate friends know that I had a problem.

As I grew older and provisionally more sophisticated, I came across theories that seemed to offer an explanation or at least an interpretation of my seizure, notably the popularized Freudianism that was so inescapable in the fifties and sixties. For a long time I adopted the view that my silly grin was psychosomatic in origin and I could get to the bottom of it, and perhaps cure it, only through psychoanalysis. Before I could explore this possibility, however, I was persuaded by a medical doctor in whom I confided (a) that the seizure was probably a kind of epilepsy and (b) that my means of coping with it were probably as sound as anything formal medicine could supply.

Like many others in the 1960s, I repeatedly came into contact with marihuana, but for several years I resisted the temptation to smoke it. I was highly visible as an SDS national officer and felt obliged to avoid bringing the organization into disrepute; besides, SDS had taken a strong anti-marihuana position at my urging. Finally, unlike most rank-and-file members of the movement, I was a family man and the father of three children toward whom I felt a parent's normal responsibilities as those were understood in the American 1950s.

But in 1970 or thereabouts, with SDS destroyed, leadership of the antiwar movement in other hands, and my paternal pretensions the victims of divorce and separation, my curiosity won out and I began to experiment with marihuana in social situations. I soon discovered that my seizures vanished when I was high. After a few puffs, the aura and its ascent to the dreaded rictus simply did not occur for two to three hours.

I also enjoyed the pleasures of the marihuana high itself. In sharp contradistinction to alcohol, it was no threat to self-control, and in fact improved my ability to speak extemporaneously. That alone would never have led me to become a regular user, since I was always unhappy about the idea of smoking. But marihuana's power to eliminate my seizures led me to adopt it as a regular medication. Several months ago I resolved to abandon this form of self-medication and simply suffer the consequences— more tolerable to me now than in 1970 because I am much less often called upon to speak in public (I still give perhaps a dozen public lectures a year). Nevertheless, the return of the seizures is saddening and to a certain extent dispiriting, so I have sought professional medical help in the hope of finding a workable, safe, and legal alternative.

Gordon Hanson is a fifty-three-year-old man who suffers both from grand mal epilepsy and from absence attacks. These were partially controlled with the standard drugs phenytoin (Dilantin®), primidone (Mysoline®), and phenobarbital, but there were serious side effects. Here is his account:

Thinking back to the years before high school graduation is much easier for me than thinking about what happened after that chilly day in September 1956. Northerly winds scattered the fallen leaves as I hurried to fill my bucket with bright red cranberries against the setting sun of a shorter day. My emotions were mixed; this was my first season free of school, but I was uncertain of the future.

Arriving home for supper was a pleasant experience for both me and my faithful fox terrier. Living in Minnesota was a blessing nearly missed. I was the youngest of eight children born in 1938 to turn-of-the-century Scandinavian immigrants. Mother was forty-nine at the time, and my youngest brother was nine. Life's many images of love were abundant even though material things were not. My father, like our neighbors, provided a modest income from his small dairy farm. On that September evening I felt very sleepy and retired before 10:00 P.M. Awakening was a revolving point of confusion and depression followed by nausea, headache, and muscle soreness that seemed to cover my entire body. My family surrounded the bed, their faces filled with concern. As soon as daylight came I was hurried to see our family doctor in Baudette. His diagnosis made me feel even more frightened and frustrated. How could I have epilepsy?

The affliction was kept as much a secret as possible. As the years passed, unpredictable petit mal seizures made an appearance, while the less frequent grand mal continued its haunting signs of approach—sounds of no meaning or apparent source, inability to speak, and finally the creeping paralysis that slowly engulfed my body. Unconsciousness would hide any injury until I once again regained my senses. Burns and broken bones were not uncommon, yet not as foreboding as the lingering deep depression.

Combinations of prescription drugs, including Dilantin, Mysoline, and phenobarbital, did decrease the number of seizures but definitely did not cure the problems. Deep sadness would often overwhelm my life for days. Epilepsy was naturally assumed to be the cause—no one ever told me then that the drugs used to prevent seizures also had bad side effects. I drank alcohol for a few years, but it proved to be such a short-lived escape. Finally I met a girl I wanted to marry, but because I was afraid she would reject me, I did not tell her of my epileptic problems before our marriage.

Our youth and her gift of a daughter shielded us from pain for a short time. But the necessities of survival became ever more difficult to obtain, and the seizures became more frequent. My wife began to use alcohol to hide herself from a person she had now begun to fear because of the strange seizures and lingering mood swings that created a Jekyll-Hyde syndrome. Her drinking and my response to it increased our unhappiness, which was relieved only for a short time by the births of another daughter and son in the early sixties. My seizures and financial problems increased.

At the end of the sixties I had many confrontations with the law. In the early seventies the children were temporarily removed from our home. The court told me to consult a marriage counselor, who suggested I might try marihuana to decrease the depressive effect of phenobarbital and still control the seizures. This seemed absurd to me, as my attitude was the same as the majority's: this was a drug only whispered about, definitely evil!

Thank God, I began to read about the plant and also made inquiries to other sources, including the University of Minnesota. I found out that it had been used medically in centuries gone by, and I began to smoke it regularly.

By 1976 I cut my dose of phenobarbital, Dilantin, and Mysoline by about 50 percent. Seizures had become less frequent and mood swings had dwindled, at least when marihuana was available. In 1976 I was arrested for possession of a small amount, and after that I found it harder to purchase. The judge asked me to consult a doctor. The doctor didn't deny the medical usefulness of marihuana, but because it was illegal, he suggested I take Valium. In nearly two years I took two Valium pills a day, but it made a walking zombie of me, and I still had blackouts.

In 1978 my wife was hospitalized for three days after she mistook phenobarbital for aspirin while intoxicated. That made me discard my remaining phenobarbital and Valium completely. My mind was clear after withdrawal. I decided to try growing plants from accumulated seed that spring. It was rather successful. With each new year came new methods for better quality, leaving un-

pleasant memories behind. By 1982 I was growing enough in
my garden to reduce my use of prescription drugs even further.
Grand mal seizures had vanished, and the petit mal seizures
numbered fewer than ten a year. Unfortunately, that summer I
found the law frowning on my harvest of the herb, and I was
arrested for possession of what they called a large amount. I continued to grow plants while awaiting the outcome of a long court
battle that ended in 1985 with a two-month jail sentence. I was
given more pills, but I still had seizures in jail. Another drug,
Tranxene [clorazepate, an anti-anxiety drug and muscle relaxant
related to Valium] was prescribed, but I used very little because
I realized that the effects were similar to those of Valium.

On release I again started to use marihuana for relief from the
pills and the blackouts. Our family life became pleasant as the
years slipped gently by. An average growth of forty hemp plants
supplied by nature decreased my need for man-made chemicals
to one dose of Dilantin and one dose of Mysoline a day. Petit
mal seizures now occurred five times a year or fewer, mostly in
winter when I ran out of marihuana. Life became much more
harmonious.

In 1988 there was a drought, my marihuana was stunted, and
I was forced to buy off the street only four months after harvest. The street price had risen so high I could barely afford
it. Friends helped me until the next growing season, but I still
had many seizures when marihuana was unavailable. Determined
not to be caught short again, in 1989 I planted three times as
many marihuana plants, each trimmed to resemble a short bushy
tomato plant.

In late July I pulled up a couple and put them in our old vacant
barn to dry. The rest of the story is a disaster—five police officers kicking in my front door before 6:00 A.M. and holding my
wife, my son, and myself at gunpoint. My son lost his job because he wasn't allowed to leave for work that morning. Needless
to say, all the marihuana was taken. After paying a bond, I was
released, only to relive the experience in my dreams each night

for weeks. My life since that day has been an experiment that resolves my doubts about the medical value of marihuana. Because of its unavailability I have suffered nearly two hundred seizures, including several of the grand mal type.

On June 22, 1991, what I had feared happened. A telephone call from my attorney in Minneapolis informed me that I had to report to Roseau County Jail for a sentence of six months. The Minnesota Supreme Court had denied my appeal. Now I sit in a cell with no provisions for personal safety. The cell is isolated. I have no way to communicate with the jailer's office, and the two prisoners I share it with have not been told what to do if a seizure should occur.

It is strange to think back to the early seventies, when I was told to consult a marriage counselor who advised me to use marihuana instead of prescription drugs. Now the law has taken me away from my wife and put me in prison because I complied with that suggestion, which had been successful in controlling my seizures and bringing love back to us. Now the law is once more forcing prescription drugs on me. I fear the dreaded cumulative side effects will return and cause me to become that nightmarish creature who brought so much grief to my wife and family. I cannot expect her to accept such a situation again after the solution we achieved by discovering God's creation of such a wondrous healing herb. Apparently my only alternative is to use no drugs at all when I am released. This will cause much unnecessary hardship not only for me but also for my wife, who will have to contend with the seizures and the depressive moods that follow. I can only pray that our government will recognize marihuana's medical uses before my release. If not, I cannot expect Connie to accept me home.

MULTIPLE SCLEROSIS

Multiple sclerosis (MS) is a disorder in which patches of myelin (the protective covering of nerve fibers) in the brain and spinal cord are destroyed and the normal functioning of the nerve fibers them-selves is interrupted. It seems to be an autoimmune response in which the body's defense system treats the myelin as a foreign invader. The symptoms usually appear in early adulthood, then come and go unpredictably for years. Attacks last from weeks to months, and re-mission is often incomplete, with gradual deterioration and eventual severe disability. Injury, infection, or stress may cause a relapse. The average survival time is thirty years, but some patients deteriorate much faster, and others stabilize after a few attacks.

The symptoms depend on which part of the central nervous system is affected by demyelination. Because the brain and spinal cord con-trol the entire body, the effects may appear almost anywhere. Some common symptoms are tingling, numbness, impaired vision, diffi-culty in speaking, painful muscle spasms, loss of coordination and balance (ataxia), fatigue, weakness or paralysis, tremors, loss of blad-der control, urinary tract infections, constipation, skin ulcerations, and severe depression.

No effective treatment is known. Corticosteroids, especially adrenocorticotropic hormone (ACTH) and prednisone, provide some relief for the acute symptoms, but they also produce weight gain and sometimes cause mental disturbances. The drugs most commonly used to treat muscle spasms are diazepam (Valium®), baclofen (Liore-sal®), and dantrolene (Dantrium®). Diazepam and other drugs in the benzodiazepine class, which must be given in large doses, cause drowsiness and can be addictive. Both dantrolene and baclofen are of marginal medical utility. Baclofen is a sedative and sometimes causes dizziness, weakness, or confusion. Dantrolene is a last resort because of potentially lethal liver damage; it also has a variety of other side effects, including drowsiness, dizziness, weakness, general mal-aise, abdominal cramps, diarrhea, speech and visual disturbances, seizures, headaches, impotence, tachycardia, erratic blood pressure, clinical depression, myalgia, feelings of suffocation, and confusion. Understandably, many patients cannot tolerate the immediate side effects of the standard drugs or become concerned about the long-term effects.

The use of marihuana in multiple sclerosis is illustrated in this account by Greg Paufler, a thirty-seven-year-old resident of upstate New York:

In 1973 I noticed a feeling of numbness in my left thumb that began to spread to the rest of my left hand. I explained the symptoms to a doctor, who diagnosed my problem as neuritis, said it would clear up in a few days, and recommended vitamin supplements. Within a week the numbness was gone, but I began to have difficulty maintaining my balance and sometimes had trouble walking.

By the early spring of 1974, my health was much worse, although I continued to take my vitamins. My stumbling and falling became an office joke at the insurance company where I worked as a salesman. Other employees would laughingly ask me if I had been drinking. My supervisor complained that I was seeing fewer clients and writing fewer orders. I told him that the numbness in my legs interfered with driving a car and that I was finding it increasingly difficult to write (I did not reveal that I was barely able to write at all). He did not seem satisfied with these explanations. Soon afterward a co-worker and close friend persuaded me to obtain a second opinion. As I walked into the doctor's waiting room, I fell flat on my face and cut my knee. The nurse helped me into the office. I tried to stand on my own and fell again. I told the doctor that I had sharp spasms and numbness in my legs and could not tell where my feet were without looking at them. The doctor, a general practitioner, insisted that I be hospitalized immediately, despite my protests; he said I might have a brain tumor.

I remained in the hospital for seven days of observation and medical tests supervised by a team of physicians headed by a neurologist. During this time I lost all control over my limbs and experienced severe, painful spasms. My arms and legs became numb. I could no longer walk. I was given intravenous injections of ACTH, a powerful steroid, but it didn't help; it only kept me awake and increased my appetite dramatically. On the day of my release, the supervising neurologist told me I was suffering from multiple sclerosis. He said there was no cure, but drugs like ACTH could slow its progress. He then told me to go home and get plenty of rest. He made an appointment to see me in his office—an appointment that, as it turned out, I could not keep because I was too weak to make the trip. Instead the doctor had a nurse come to our home and show my wife how to inject me with ACTH.

Shortly after I returned home, and while I was bedridden, some friends came to visit and we smoked a few marihuana cigarettes. Afterward I felt better, but attributed that effect to the mild "high." My spasms also became less severe, but I gave the daily injections of ACTH credit for that. Despite some improvement, I remained bedridden and soon began to feel the effects of chronic high-dose steroid therapy. I retained fluids and became bloated; I gained a hundred pounds in six weeks because ACTH made me ravenously hungry. I had sleepless nights. I started losing my concentration. My mental attitude was dismal and I became depressed. After three months of intensive therapy, my condition had barely improved. I could walk only when supported by my wife and a cane or walker.

The doctor told me I had to take ACTH for another three months, but he was obviously concerned about the side effects. He warned me of the danger of a sudden heart attack or respiratory failure. To reduce fluid retention, he prescribed a powerful diuretic, which he acknowledged could cause kidney stones or death from kidney failure. The steroid therapy was still not working, and its adverse effects became worse. My weight rose from 170 pounds before taking ACTH to 300 pounds within several weeks after starting the second round of ACTH therapy. Breathing became difficult as fluids pressed against my lungs. My feet and legs were swollen. None of my clothes fit. I developed severe, intense depression marked by abrupt mood shifts. I would become profoundly upset for no reason; I would suddenly start to cry or have violent thoughts. After six months I felt that I had lost all control over my life. On rare, very good days I could shuffle across my bedroom by leaning against the wall and using my wife and a walker for support. Even then I could not maintain my balance or support my weight, and I often fell. Most of the time I was bedridden. My spasms continued, and my limbs were out of control.

At the end of the sixth month, I saw my doctor again and told him my condition was getting worse. He said that my MS was very severe and had progressed very rapidly; only ACTH could help. He recommended another three months and increased the dose by 50 percent. He also prescribed a sleeping pill and Valium to reduce my spasms. I agreed to give ACTH another try, but changed my mind a couple of days later. I could not take it any longer. If the only choice was MS or this treatment, I would rather have the MS. When I stopped taking ACTH, my vision became blurred and I had episodes of tunnel vision. I could not focus and lost my ability to read; the MS was attacking me in an entirely different way. My doctor became very worried and immediately prescribed prednisone, a powerful oral steroid. Again I received little therapeutic benefit but there were many adverse effects, this time even more intense; in less than a month I gained more than eighty pounds. But there was worse to come. Although I did not know it, the steroids were stripping my body of critically important potassium.

One day, while sitting in my living room, I realized I could not talk. I was semicatatonic. One of my children walked up and spoke to me. I heard her but could not see her and could not respond, except by crying. My wife and daughter immediately took me to a hospital emergency room. I have no memory of the trip and did not know where I was when we arrived. I remember being slumped in a chair alone, then surrounded by nearly a dozen doctors and nurses, all frantically talking. They asked me questions I am not sure I heard. When I tried to respond I could not speak. Medical records indicate that I nearly died that day; my body had almost no potassium in it. I was given massive injections and an oral potassium supplement.

This experience caused me to become deeply disenchanted with drugs, doctors, and hospitals. I stopped taking all steroids, although I continued to use Valium and other mood-altering drugs. Unable to walk, read, or be with my family, I began smoking marihuana to relieve the boredom, four to six joints a day. One evening some old friends came to visit and we smoked several joints. When they rose to leave I stood up to say goodbye. Everyone in the room suddenly stopped talking and stared at me. I realized that I had spontaneously stood unassisted, as if it were perfectly natural.

I was stunned. My wife and our friends were stunned. I took a few unassisted steps before my legs, weak from atrophy, gave out. I had walked! I wondered if it was the marihuana, and asked my doctor, who dismissed the idea and insisted that marihuana had no beneficial effect on MS. My wife, too, was skeptical, but I kept on experimenting. I soon discovered that when I did not smoke marihuana my spasms were more frequent and intense. When I smoked it, my condition stabilized, then dramatically improved. I could walk unaided, and my vision was less blurred. But my doctor and my wife remained skeptical. In what I now realize was a foolish attempt to prove to others what I already knew to be true, I decided to stop smoking marihuana for six months.

As soon as I stopped I began to lose what I had gained. I had severe spasms in my back muscles. After four months I had lost control of my hands, arms, feet, and legs. My dose of Valium rose to 120 mg daily, and I began to realize that I was chemically dependent, an addict. I stopped taking Valium and suffered a severe withdrawal reaction from this "safe," "medically accepted" drug. I lost all interest in life; I was sleepless, restless, and constantly agitated; I fell into a dark depression; my mood shifts became even more erratic and pronounced; my spasms became intensely painful.

When I could no longer sit up, much less walk, I resumed

smoking marihuana daily. Within a few weeks I was able to walk again unaided. I was soon walking half a block alone with some effort. I regained strength as I got more exercise, and my eyesight returned to normal. After six months all my symptoms had improved greatly. The spasms had vanished, and I had regained the ability to read, write, and walk. One evening I went out with my children and, for the first time in two years, showed them how to kick a soccer ball. I could kick a ball! I felt reborn.

But I was still uncertain whether marihuana was responsible. Marihuana was something I used for fun, a social drug. I did not believe that such a simple and safe drug could produce such a startling improvement. It was all the easier to ignore the obvious because my doctor and my wife continued to laugh at the idea. To show myself that it was not really the marihuana that was helping, I decided to stop smoking yet again. At first gradually and then more rapidly, the muscle spasms returned. Within a few weeks I needed a cane, then a walker. Eventually I was bedridden again. After four months I decided to start smoking again. My condition immediately stabilized, then began to improve. I was happy but very confused. This pattern continued. I would smoke marihuana until my condition improved, then stop. For reasons I cannot explain, I found it hard to believe that marihuana was really the cause of these dramatic changes in my health.

In 1980 my brother showed me a newspaper article about an MS patient in Washington named Sam Diana who had convinced a court of law that his use of marihuana was a "medical necessity." I was astonished to learn that I was not the only MS patient getting relief from marihuana. It was even more astonishing that doctors, researchers, and other MS patients had supported Mr. Diana's claim and the court had ruled in his favor. I no longer felt the need to prove to myself or anyone else that marihuana was helpful; I started listening to my body and went back to smoking regularly.

For the past seven years my MS has been well controlled, except when I run out of marihuana and cannot find or afford more.

Most MS patients grow progressively weaker and more crippled; I have improved. I can stand on one foot with my eyes closed. I walk completely unaided. I can actually run! This may seem insignificant to someone who has never been bedridden, crippled, and unable to move or speak, but to me it is a miracle. On top of all that, marihuana allows me to maintain an erection long enough to complete the sex act. I have never become chemically dependent on marihuana, and I have no withdrawal symptoms when I stop smoking. Compared to the steroids, tranquilizers, and sedatives usually prescribed for MS patients, marihuana is remarkably safe and benign.

My doctor is amazed by the improvement in my symptoms. On a scale of one to 100, he rates my physical and mental health at 95. He no longer insists that marihuana is useless. At the end of our last meeting he looked me in the eye and told me to keep doing whatever it is I am doing, because it works.

I do not like breaking the law. I do not enjoy paying terribly inflated prices to drug dealers for an unregulated, uncontrolled product. But I do like to walk, talk, read, write, and see. My doctor and I are now exploring the possibility of gaining legal access to marihuana through the Food and Drug Administration's "Compassionate IND" program, despite the extraordinarily slow and complicated procedure required.

Most MS patients in the United States now learn about marihuana through support groups or the grapevine. Many anecdotes testify to its capacity to relieve tremors and loss of muscle coordination. Neurologists often hear about it from their patients. Yet the medical literature includes only a few cases like the following one, reported in 1983:

A 30-year-old man had a ten-year history of MS consisting of exacerbations and remissions, resulting in paraparesis, diplopia, ataxia, numbness and parasthesia in all extremities, urinary retention, incontinence, and impotence. Medical treatments had included ACTH, corticosteroids, and azathioprine. A disabling tremor had been a consistent problem for more than a year. The tremor was maximal in the head and neck and resulted in particular problems while eating, because it increased as efforts were made to put food in the mouth. The tremor was diminished, but not abolished, when the patient was supine with his head fully supported. It disappeared with sleep. Treatment with diazepam, alcohol, propranolol, and physostigmine were uniformly unsuccessful. Marihuana had been used to control the tremor on an almost daily basis for at least one year prior to this study without evidence of diminishing response. The initial 5 mg dose of THC resulted in a decrease in head and neck tremor within 30 to 60 minutes which lasted approximately six hours. The dose resulted in a very mild "high" which did not appear to impair judgment. Mild hand ataxia seen in finger-nose-finger testing was little changed, but the patient's ability to write was considerably improved [see fig. 1], and his use of eating utensils was markedly improved. When placebo capsules were substituted no improvement occurred in spite of a "high" sensation. Repeated testing with the active drug on two occasions again demonstrated the response.[14]

Another recent report was published by neurologists at the University of Göttingen in Germany, who noticed that one of their patients, a thirty-year-old man with multiple sclerosis, used smoked marihuana to treat his motor and sexual handicaps. They tested him with clinical ratings, electromyographic study of his leg reflexes, and electromagnetic recording of his hand tremors (fig. 2). Their conclusion was that cannabis warranted further evaluation as a treatment for both muscle spasms and ataxia (loss of coordination).[15]

Debbi Talshir is a thirty-nine-year-old divorced woman who has treated her multiple sclerosis with cannabis for fourteen years. She tells her story:

14. D. B. Clifford, "Tetrahydrocannabinol for Tremor in Multiple Sclerosis," *Annals of Neurology* 13 (1983): 669–671.

15. H. M. Meinck, P. W. Schönle, and B. Conrad, "Effect of Cannabinoids on Spasticity and Ataxia in Multiple Sclerosis," *Journal of Neurology* 236 (1989): 120–122.

CONTROL   THC 5 MG

TREMOR RECORDING-HEAD

1 sec

Figure 1. Handwriting sample and movement artifact from head, recorded before and ninety minutes after ingestion of 5 mg of tetrahydrocannabinol. Reproduced from D. B. Clifford, "Tetrahydracannabinol for Tremor in Multiple Sclerosis," *Annals of Neurology* 13 (1983): 669–671.

before

after

10 cm

700 ms

Figure 2. Electromagnetic recording of the finger and hand action tremor in a pointing task on the morning before and in the evening after smoking a marihuana cigarette. Reproduced from H. M. Meinck, P. W. Schönle, and B. Conrad, "Effect of Cannabinoids on Spasticity and Ataxia in Multiple Sclerosis," *Journal of Neurology* 236 (1989): 120–122.

I was diagnosed with multiple sclerosis in 1977. One of its first symptoms was optic neuropathy. The optic nerve connects the brain and eye, and optic neuropathy is a degeneration of that connection. It can cause partial blindness. First a big cloud appeared in my vision and I could not see so well; the cloud then became black in the right eye.

For the neuropathy I was given ACTH. I gained about 100 pounds because I retained water and my appetite increased dramatically (I was always starving). The ACTH also caused mood swings that made me intolerable to my co-workers and friends. Even I was frightened by them. Finally they subsided, only to return a year and a half later, along with the optic neuropathy. This time a co-worker recommended marihuana and I smoked a couple of cigarettes daily. I didn't gain weight or have mood swings, and the optic neuropathy subsided in three weeks.

As the MS progressed, I was given Lioresal (baclofen) for muscle spasms. Yes, it caused side effects: drowsiness and just general lethargy. I found that marihuana stopped the spasms and relaxed my muscles, but not so much that they became useless. My neurologist at Massachusetts General Hospital, where I was first diagnosed, and my current neurologist here on Cape Cod know that I use marihuana to manage those symptoms and others. It is on my record, but they won't [cannot] supply legal prescriptions—very disheartening, but understandable in the present climate of the drug war. Since 1980 I have been confined to a wheelchair. I cannot eat unless I smoke some marihuana first; it relaxes the sphincter muscles in my stomach and esophagus. My loss of appetite is profound, but if I smoke a marihuana cigarette I am relaxed and can hold food down. Often I have difficulty breathing. I don't understand why smoking anything would relax the breathing mechanisms, but marihuana does.

To me, marihuana is essential. I don't shake any more, I can eat, I can breathe. It even has a very good effect on my neurogenic bladder—a neurological disorder in which a person loses control of the sphincter muscles of the bladder. If there is even a drop of urine in the bladder, the sphincter muscles go into spasm and you lose urine. Marihuana doesn't cure it, but it helps. I generally smoke five marihuana cigarettes a day.

I am very angry that I have to deal with people whom I wouldn't ordinarily socialize with, such as drug dealers. I also have to save my pennies if I am going to get any marihuana, and it is getting increasingly difficult to find. I find myself running around, making phone calls, and spending most of my time looking for it.

A patient whose loss of muscle coordination proved to be an early symptom of multiple sclerosis was brought to our attention by her psychiatrist. For several years he had been trying to get her to give up the habit of smoking a small amount of marihuana at bedtime to defeat her chronic insomnia. After persuading her to stop, he sought advice from us when he realized that the cannabis had been suppressing the symptoms of her previously undiagnosed multiple sclerosis; ataxia appeared when she stopped smoking and disappeared when she started again. He was concerned because he thought marihuana was highly toxic; our assurances that it was not relieved that fear. His patient tells her story:

> I had finally gotten where I wanted to be. What I lacked in education I had made up for with hard work, long hours, and the boss that every young businesswoman dreams of. Starting at twenty-one as the lowest-paid clerk in a small local company, I was now, at forty-five, a finance executive for a billion-dollar electronics firm.
>
> The work was hard, fast, and demanding, but very satisfying. Stepping the pace down at the end of the day was difficult, and I found that smoking a very small amount of marihuana at bedtime allowed me to relax and get to sleep. By 1986 I had been smoking for about fifteen years and wasn't concerned that such a small amount could be harmful.
>
> From 1986 through 1989 I fought a continuing low-key battle with my psychiatrist about this. I felt that my experience was entirely positive and that any ill effects would have become evident in fifteen years. My doctor, however, thought I should not use an untested and, incidentally, illegal drug.
>
> In October 1989 I agreed to replace marihuana with Desyrel [trazodone, an antidepressant with sedative properties]. Although it was not as effective, and I had hangovers the morning after, the substitution seemed acceptable for a few days. On the sixth morning, however, I realized that I had lost most of my ability to balance. I could barely stand upright or walk without support. While driving to the doctor's office, I also found that what I call my auto-pilot had been wiped clean. Activities normally performed subconsciously, like driving, now required

conscious thought. I even had to relearn the way the key turned to unlock the car. I was also more tired than I had ever been before.

In the next six weeks I took no drugs at all, not even an aspirin, while doctors tested me for every disease known to Western medicine. During this time my symptoms did not improve. After the tests I received the devastating news that I had multiple sclerosis, an incurable nerve disease with little hope of meaningful treatment. Although I had been told that MS symptoms come and go without warning, I was disturbed by the apparent coincidence and hesitantly raised the marihuana question with a neurologist. I was given an angry lecture and instructions to return only when I could pass a drug screening test.

I couldn't let it go at that. Logic dictated that I at least try smoking marihuana. My doctor [psychiatrist] was still opposed, but did express some interest in what might happen, so I decided to start. About a week later I noticed an improvement, and a few weeks later I was able to return to work at about 85 percent of normal.

The improvement could have been spontaneous—MS is very capricious—but I wasn't about to take a chance, and I went on smoking until the spring of 1990, when I ran out of marihuana and was unable to get any more. A week later all my symptoms were again severe.

My doctors still thought it was a coincidence, but I didn't. I began a nationwide search for supplies of marihuana and for a neurologist who would at least listen to my story with an open mind. I found the marihuana, but not the neurologist. Since it is illegal to conduct experiments with marihuana, there is no scientific evidence of its value; and, because there is no scientific evidence of its value, the government will not allow experimentation.

When I finally received some marihuana from a friend and resumed smoking, I only returned to 60 percent of normal and could work only at home. Later in 1990 the entire sequence was

repeated, and this time I returned to less than 50 percent of normal. I could no longer work more than half an hour at a time.
Early in 1991 I was retired at 100 percent disability.

I still have a small supply of marihuana, and am afraid of what
will happen when it runs out. Meanwhile I am searching for a
neurologist who will apply for a Compassionate IND, and I am
praying that the laws can be changed.

There are hints in this case and others that cannabis not only relieves the symptoms of multiple sclerosis—muscle spasms, tremor,
loss of muscle coordination (ataxia) and bladder control, insomnia—
but also retards the progression of the disease. Multiple sclerosis is
a disorder caused by an immune system gone haywire; current treatments include the use of steroids that suppress immune functioning.
Although smoked marihuana apparently does not increase suscepti-
bility to infectious disease, there is evidence that THC has immuno-
suppressive effects. With this in mind, a group of investigators tested
its ability to suppress experimental autoimmune encephalitis (EAE),
a disease that has been used as a laboratory model of multiple sclerosis in guinea pigs. When animals were exposed to the disease and
then treated with a placebo, all developed severe EAE and more than
98 percent died. Animals treated with THC had either no or only
mild symptoms, and more than 95 percent survived. On inspection
the brain tissue of the animals treated with THC proved to be much
less inflamed.[16]

PARAPLEGIA AND QUADRIPLEGIA

Paraplegia is weakness or paralysis of muscles in the lower body
caused by disease or injury in the middle or lower part of the spinal
cord. If the injury is near the neck, the arms as well as the legs
are affected and quadriplegia develops. Paraplegia and quadriplegia

16. W. D. Lyman, J. R. Sonett, C. F. Brosnan, R. Elkin, and M. B. Bornstein, "Delta-
9-tetrahydrocannabinol: A Novel Treatment for Experimental Autoimmune Encephalitis," *Journal of Neuroimmunology* 23 (1989): 73–81.

are often accompanied by pain and muscle spasms; standard treatments are opioids for the pain, baclofen and diazepam for the muscle spasms. Many paraplegics and quadriplegics have now discovered that cannabis not only relieves their pain more safely than opioids but also effectively suppresses their muscle jerks and tremors. The following account by Chris Woiderski is illustrative:

In June 1989, I was twenty-seven years old and had been working as an industrial engineer for five and a half years, selling pneumatic and automation equipment to manufacturing plants and factories. I was pretty successful at it. I had used marihuana off and on for several years to relax. After a long hard day I would go home, have dinner with my girl friend, smoke some marihuana, and unwind. I usually spent evenings in my home office, and I found that smoking marihuana not only relaxed me but helped me concentrate on my work.

I would sometimes think that things just couldn't get any better for me. I had a good job, made excellent money, and lived with the woman I was going to marry in a few months. Then, in June 1989, I suffered an accidental gunshot wound. I was rushed to a hospital and wheeled into surgery. I awoke the next evening in a semi-coherent state, feeling the pain from tubes in my chest and throat. After ten days in the intensive care unit, a neurologist told me there was nothing he could do for me. Although the bullet had missed my spinal cord, swelling had left me permanently paralyzed from the chest down. When I finally realized I would never be cured, I got angry, and the anger never went away.

I was no longer able to work, so I subsisted on a meager Social Security pension. Luckily, I had served in the Navy and was eligible to receive medical supplies and care from the Veterans' Administration. After two months of watching me try to do the simplest tasks (dressing, showering, getting in and out of bed), my girl friend just couldn't take it any more and moved back to her parents' house.

Four months after my injury, I began to experience the strange and somewhat painful sensations known as muscle spasms. At first they affected only my feet and lower legs, but soon I had them in all my paralyzed muscles. I was given a drug called baclofen, but even the maximum dosage did not provide much relief. There were plenty of unpleasant side effects, though—drowsiness, severe headaches, excessive sweating, insomnia, and dry mouth.

My spasms became more and more violent. After they caused me to fall out of bed, the doctors added 20 mg a day of Valium, then another 20 mg. I was becoming a pharmacological zombie.

There were many other paralyzed patients at the V.A. hospital. Some had been paraplegics for more than twenty years. They told me they had thrown away their prescription spasm medications years ago and now used marihuana instead. They said it worked better and had far fewer side effects. I tried it. One marihuana cigarette gave me immediate relief without the debilitating side effects of Valium and baclofen. Everyday tasks like showering and dressing became remarkably easier to accomplish. Since then, whenever I can find marihuana, I smoke three to four cigarettes a day. I have few or no spasms, and I am spared the need to take twelve very toxic and addictive pills daily. I have also discovered that I can achieve an erection when I smoke marihuana; the only way I could do that before was by injecting prostaglandin directly into my penis.

About two-thirds of the paralyzed patients I've met use marihuana to control muscle spasms and pain. Present Drug Enforcement Administration regulations forbid our doctors to prescribe marihuana for us. The government is now waging a war on drugs that in effect targets me and other paralyzed patients. This is not only unreasonable and unfair, but blatantly immoral. Because we choose to use the most effective and safest drug for our condition, the government unjustly puts us in the same criminal category as heroin junkies.

I am filing an Investigational New Drug Application (IND) with the Food and Drug Administration. It is the same procedure used by several other Americans who have won the right to smoke marihuana legally for medical purposes. I hope my request will be granted. If not, I will continue to smoke marihuana anyway and risk being unjustly arrested, prosecuted, and jailed.

Chris Woiderski notes that marihuana enabled him to achieve a normal erection. One report in the medical literature confirms this effect. A thirty-year-old patient had suffered from MS for six years and was wheelchair-bound because of muscle spasms and ataxia. His erections lasted less than five minutes, and he was unable to ejaculate. When he smoked marihuana, both his motor functions and his sexual functions improved immediately. He can now sustain an erection for more than half an hour, and his sexual life is satisfactory.[17]

Once again, many patients have discovered through word of mouth or support groups a medical use of marihuana that doctors are not supposed to tell them about. The odor of marihuana smoke is said to be omnipresent on some V.A. hospital paraplegia and quadriplegia wards. A survey of forty-three persons with spinal cord injuries conducted in 1982 indicated that twenty-two of them were using marihuana for muscle spasms.[18] The percentage has probably increased in the past decade. Yet, again, very little on the subject appears in the medical literature. We have been able to find only one recent study. In 1990 three Swiss neurologists reported on the treatment of a paraplegic patient with painful spasms in both legs that were being constantly medicated with baclofen, clonazepam (an anti-anxiety drug related to Valium), and codeine for pain. The experiment took place in two stages. In the first stage the patient took oral THC instead of codeine fourteen times over a period of three months. In the second phase he was given either 5 mg of oral THC, 50 mg of oral codeine, or a placebo. The three experimental conditions were each applied eighteen times in the course of five months. He continued to take baclofen

17. Meinck, Schönle, and Conrad, "Effect of Cannabinoids."
18. J. Malec, R. F. Harvey, and J. J. Cayner, "Cannabis Effect on Spasticity in Spinal Cord Injury," *Archives of Physical and Medical Rehabilitation* 63 (March 1982): 116–118.

and clonazepam throughout the experiment. As compared with placebo, both codeine and THC improved the quality of sleep, and both produced an analgesic effect, but only THC reduced muscle spasms. Both THC and codeine also improved the patient's bladder control, mood, and ability to concentrate on intellectual work. Since THC was as good as codeine in most respects and better at preventing muscle spasms, the neurologists concluded that it should be considered in the treatment of paraplegics.[19]

AIDS

The American AIDS epidemic first came to notice in 1981, when five homosexual men in Los Angeles were found to have developed a mysterious and profound immune deficiency that was being exploited by opportunistic infections (microorganisms that are normally harmless but become dangerous when the immune system is impaired). In 1984 the human immunodeficiency virus (HIV) was found to be the cause of AIDS. By now more than 150,000 Americans have died of the disease; nearly 2 million are infected with the virus, and perhaps as many as a quarter of a million are ill. Although the spread of AIDS has slowed among homosexuals, the reservoir is so huge that the number of cases is sure to grow. Women and children as well as both heterosexual and homosexual men are now being affected; the disease is spreading most rapidly among inner-city black and Hispanic intravenous drug abusers and their sexual partners.

The period of incubation (between infection and the development of symptoms) is variable but averages eight to ten years. It appears that almost all infected persons will eventually become ill. No cure is known. Opportunistic infections and neoplasms (cancerous growths) can be treated in standard ways, and the virus itself can be attacked with antiviral drugs, of which the best known is zidovudine (AZT).

19. M. Maurer, V. Henn, A. Dittrich, and A. Hofmann, "Delta-9-tetrahydrocannabinol Shows Antispastic and Analgesic Effects in a Single Case Double-blind Trial," *European Archives of Psychiatry and Clinical Neuroscience* 240 (1990): 1–4.

Unfortunately, AZT suppresses the production of red blood cells by the bone marrow, decreases the number of white blood cells, and has many damaging effects on the digestive system. It sometimes causes severe nausea that heightens the danger of semi-starvation for patients who are already suffering from nausea and losing weight because of the illness.

Ron Mason, age thirty-three, tells his story:

October 19, 1983, was the day I found out I had hepatitis B. For some time I had been noticing a full-page ad in *Gay Chicago* magazine, but I avoided reading it because it looked too depressing (it was a picture of a man in a hospital bed being fed intravenously). When I finally broke down and read it, I found that it was an open letter to the gay community from the Liver Foundation in New Jersey. It said that two-thirds of gay men, whether they knew it or not, were contracting hepatitis B (this was back before "safe sex") at one time or another. Fifty percent of people who are infected with the virus have symptoms, some mild, some severe. Ninety percent develop antibodies after an infection and are no longer susceptible; 10 percent become carriers, and 2 percent die. A vaccine was available, the ad said. So the next time I was at the gay VD clinic, I asked the clerk to screen me for antibodies. It turned out that I had the infection itself. It was too late for vaccination. Now I knew why I was nauseous, often threw up, and tired so easily. Although I lacked appetite, the doctor told me I had to eat. Since I had a liver disease, I naturally gave up drinking (I had never drunk much anyway), and now began to smoke more marihuana. I noticed that my appetite increased dramatically after smoking. I began to smoke daily and gained weight rapidly. Two years later I had not yet produced antibodies and was officially designated a hepatitis carrier.

December 23, 1986, is a day I will remember the rest of my life, the day I took the HIV test and found that I had the virus. The huge purplish red marks on my legs, I was to learn, resulted from internal bleeding caused by HIV infection. HIV was also the cause of my severe psoriasis.

In April 1984 I was referred by doctors at a gay VD clinic to what was later to become known as the AIDS clinic in Chicago. I saw doctors there for seven years and gained 40 pounds, achieving normal weight. The doctors knew I smoked marihuana and did not forbid it, although they urged moderation. I cannot tolerate AZT because of anemia. All the other antiviral drugs are damaging to my hepatitis-infected liver.

Three years ago one of my doctors told me that I am one of a handful of people who have been going to the clinic for several years and are not dead or gravely ill; the doctors don't know why. I attribute part of my success to smoking marihuana. It makes me feel as if I am living with AIDS rather than just existing. My appetite returns, and once I have eaten, I don't feel sick anymore. Marihuana improves my state of mind, and that makes me feel better physically.

I have almost died twice from allergic reactions to Compound Q, an extract of the wild Chinese cucumber root that destroys infected immune cells. Compound Q is illegal, but the government chooses to look the other way. Why can't it do the same for marihuana? Both drugs are illegal and both are used to treat AIDS patients. One will get you in trouble, and the other will not. What a joke!

In the spring of 1990, I was arrested in suburban Chicago for possession of marihuana and my car was impounded. I have not only lost my medicine but find it difficult to travel to the AIDS clinic in downtown Chicago. My appetite is no longer what it used to be; I have lost fourteen pounds, tire more easily, and sometimes become so run down I feel as though I am going to be sick. I am taking Prozac [fluoxetine, an antidepressant] prescribed by a suburban doctor who knows virtually nothing about AIDS or hepatitis B. I am very depressed and have contemplated suicide several times.

I have had to get cash advances totaling three thousand dollars on my credit card to pay legal fees for two court cases. The felony charge has been dismissed, and I am now trying to get my auto back (the federal civil case) so that I can go to the AIDS clinic.

My lawyer tells me I may succeed. Even if I do, how can I relieve the nausea and stimulate my appetite so that I feel better? I tried Marinol and it had no effect. What am I supposed to do? Nothing? If the only way I can stay healthy is to smoke marihuana and therefore feel good enough to eat, why can't I? I wish the government would stop being so hypocritical and let me do what I need to do to live the rest of my days as comfortably as possible.

A predecessor of AIDS is AIDS-related complex, or ARC. Its symptoms include swelling of the lymph nodes, fever, nausea, diarrhea, pain, and fatigue. ARC may persist for a long time or progress quickly to AIDS. When "Dr. Z," a physician with ARC, began AZT therapy about two years ago, his CBC, T-cell counts, LFTs (liver function tests), and other immune measures stabilized. Unfortunately, he also began to suffer from severe nausea and diarrhea (eight to twelve stools per day). His personal physician prescribed promethazine and prochlorperazine for nausea; kaolin, diphenoxylate with atropine, loperamide, and ranitidine for diarrhea and a hyperactive gastrointestinal tract. None of these drugs gave adequate relief. Dr. Z then discovered that small amounts of cannabis smoked throughout the day eliminated the nausea entirely and reduced the number of stools to two or three a day, without the use of any other drugs. He had also been suffering from severe fatigue that interfered with many everyday activities. Cannabis reduced this fatigue as well. His account follows:

> Because of the rabid hysteria that has infected the United States in regard to AIDS and the drug war, I have chosen to remain anonymous. I am a physician with ARC who believes that marihuana is the best single drug to alleviate many of the maladies associated with AIDS. Some preliminary information will place this discussion in proper perspective. Like many others, I first experimented with marihuana in college. I enjoyed the experience, but a pre-med student at a respected Ivy League college had little time for such recreation. In all, I probably smoked fewer than a dozen times in college. Medical school, internship, and residency followed without further marihuana use. I then set up

a practice in the small town where I still live, although I am no longer practicing medicine.

About two years ago I was diagnosed with ARC. My symptoms included fatigue, headaches, severe leg cramps, nausea, and occasional sweats. AZT did little to improve any of the symptoms, and even made the nausea worse, but it did slow the progress of the disease. I had a medicine cabinet filled with barbiturates and narcotics, all potent legal Class [Schedule] II drugs, for my pain and discomfort. Although these drugs helped, they often left me even more fatigued and lethargic. The pills I took for my leg pains left my intestinal tract tied up in knots. This, coupled with the nausea caused by AZT, necessitated another pill, an antiemetic. All in all, between the pills, the pain, and the nausea, it was not a lifestyle that made me look forward to starting a new day.

I continued "living" this way until I was invited to a party with friends I had not seen for some time. I was quite reluctant to go, since I had the usual throbbing headache and leg cramps, but I felt I needed to socialize. Someone brought out some grass, and soon I found myself headache-free and with only the mildest of leg discomfort. I couldn't believe it—pain-free without the side effects of the narcotics. In fact, I felt better than at any time since I had been diagnosed. Trust me, I was not in a semi-comatose state either. I was no more relaxed than after a couple of socially acceptable martinis.

Wondering whether there was some real basis to my discovery, I spoke to other people with AIDS about marihuana. Almost unanimously, they said it made them feel better. Unfortunately, given the current U.S. policy, most (including myself) do not want to risk litigation and exposure. It is tragic enough to face the diagnosis of AIDS, but compounding the problem with criminal charges would be unbearable. So we must continue to use potent, addictive Class II narcotics and barbiturates when an illegal drug would offer better relief.

Recently I visited Amsterdam, a city where marihuana use is condoned. It is not, strictly speaking, legal, but it is not punished as a crime. Believe me, I felt as if I had been cured of AIDS. Although I had usually taken eight to twelve pills a day, I took almost none while I was there. I smoked whenever I felt the need, usually when I became nauseous or had leg cramps or headaches—two or three cigarettes a day. I was often free of symptoms most of the day, without having to worry about being arrested. I could be a responsible adult and use the drug when I felt it was necessary, as I used the pills at home. I felt truly alive once again—a rarity when you suffer from AIDS.

Unfortunately, the cure was short-lived. On returning to the United States I had to start using the legal painkillers and anti-emetics again.

Being both a physician and a patient with HIV disease has been a mixed blessing. I have seen many suffer and die and realize that that will probably be my fate as well. But I also know there is a drug, namely marihuana, that relieves at least some of the suffering and can make the life of a person with AIDS more productive. It cannot be prescribed, however, in this kinder and gentler America. This is truly UNCONSCIONABLE. At the rate the epidemic is growing, we will all know someone who is or will be afflicted with HIV. Are we such a ruthless society that we will continue to allow this government's "war on drugs" to force those so afflicted either to become criminals or to suffer needlessly?

Because marihuana is illegal, Dr. Z decided to seek a prescription for dronabinol (Marinol®). He approached his personal physician, who knew little about dronabinol and was reluctant to prescribe it for fear of "addiction" and possible "euphoria." Finally, he wrote a prescription for 5 mg a day, half the dose recommended by a representative of the company that manufactures Marinol. It has taken the general public ten years to realize how serious the HIV epidemic is. Unfortunately, it may take physicians another ten years to appreciate the options for treatment.

Doctor Z applied to four pharmacies before he found one that would fill the prescription. After a five-day wait, he obtained the prescribed dose. A five-day trial proved unhelpful. He then increased the dose on his own to 5 mg twice a day and noticed some improvement. But he soon went back to using marihuana, despite the legal penalties. Smoking allowed him to titrate the dose for a constant blood level, and illegal marihuana relieved his symptoms better than legal Marinol—a fact that is common knowledge among patients who have tried both.

The only study to date of dronabinol and AIDS has demonstrated that it is useful in patients with symptomatic HIV infection. In addition to relieving nausea, it caused significant weight gain in 70 percent of patients. However, about one-fifth of the patients discontinued taking the drug because of unpleasant psychotropic effects.[20] These results are more or less consistent with the experience with Marinol in the treatment of the nausea and vomiting that accompany cancer chemotherapy. Most of these patients preferred to use smoked cannabis, and one suspects that the same will be true with AIDS patients, just as it was in the case of Dr. Z.

The most recent addition to the anti-AIDS armamentarium is a drug called foscarnet (Foscavir®). About 20 percent of AIDS patients develop cytomegalovirus retinitis, an infectious disease of the eye that can cause blindness. Foscarnet was developed to treat this disease; in a recent study it also turned out to prolong the lives of AIDS patients considerably.[21] Unfortunately, among other serious side effects, it causes nausea. There is every reason to believe that this nausea is sensitive to cannabis. If so, and if the hopes for foscarnet pan out, there will be yet another compelling reason for people with AIDS to use marihuana.

Recreational users are familiar with the fact that marihuana is an

20. T. F. Plasse, R. W. Gorter, S. H. Krasnow, et al., "Recent Clinical Experience with Dronabinol," *Pharmacology, Biochemistry and Behavior* 40 (1991): 695–700.

21. AIDS Research Group, in collaboration with the AIDS Clinical Trials Group, "Mortality in Patients with the Acquired Immunodeficiency Syndrome Treated with Either Foscarnet or Ganciclovir for Cytomegalovirus Retinitis," *New England Journal of Medicine* 326 (1992): 213–220.

appetite stimulant. They have long been aware that it not only makes them hungrier but enhances the flavor of food and the pleasure of eating. This effect has been demonstrated experimentally more than once. In a study conducted in 1971, four groups of subjects received either marihuana extract, alcohol, dextroamphetamine, or a placebo after fasting for twelve hours. Then they were periodically offered milkshakes and asked to say how hungry they were and how much they enjoyed the food. The subjects who took marihuana felt hungrier and ate more; those who took dextroamphetamine felt less hungry and ate less; alcohol had a negligible effect.[22]

In a later study, the body weight and caloric intake of twenty-seven marihuana users and ten control subjects were compared for twenty-one days on a hospital research ward. The marihuana smokers ate more and gained weight (the controls did not). When they stopped smoking marihuana, they immediately began to eat less.[23] Marihuana's power to enhance appetite has been demonstrated again more recently. Nine subjects smoked two to three placebo cigarettes daily and then switched to marihuana cigarettes of average potency. Their food intake significantly increased, mainly because of increased snacking rather than consuming larger meals.[24]

CHRONIC PAIN

Severe chronic pain is usually treated with opioid narcotics and various synthetic analgesics, but these drugs have many limitations. Opioids are addictive, and tolerance develops; nonaddictive synthetic analgesics are often not powerful enough. One might have expected

22. L. E. Hollister, "Hunger and Appetite after Single Doses of Marihuana, Alcohol, and Dextroamphetamine," *Clinical Pharmacology and Therapeutics* 12 (January–February 1971): 44–49.

23. I. Greenberg, J. Kuehnle, J. H. Mendelson, and J. G. Bernstein, "Effects of Marihuana Use on Body Weight and Caloric Intake in Humans," *Journal of Psychopharmacology* (Berlin) 49 (1976): 79–84.

24. R. W. Foltin, J. V. Brady, and M. W. Fischman, "Behavioral Analysis of Marijuana Effects on Food Intake in Humans," *Pharmacology, Biochemistry and Behavior* 25 (1986): 577–582.

pain specialists to take a second look at cannabis, but the medical literature again suggests little reconsideration until 1975, when one of the few modern studies of cannabis for the relief of pain was conducted at the University of Iowa. Researchers there gave oral THC or a placebo at random to hospitalized cancer patients who were in severe pain. The THC relieved pain for several hours in doses as low as 5 to 10 mg, and for even longer at 20 mg. At this dose and in this setting, THC proved to be a sedative as well. It had fewer physical side effects than other commonly used analgesics.[25]

In another study conducted in 1975, codeine, THC, and placebo were compared in thirty-six patients with advanced cancer. Codeine and THC were equally effective, but some patients found the psychoactive effects of THC (20 mg, compared with 120 mg of codeine) to be uncomfortable. It should be noted that none of these patients knew what drug they were receiving; most had never used marihuana and were unprepared for the alteration in consciousness. If they had been prepared, they might not have been uncomfortable.[26]

In the same year, Canadian investigators studied the analgesic effect of smoked marihuana in normal subjects, half of whom had used cannabis before. Their tolerance for pain from pressure on a thumbnail increased significantly after they smoked marihuana, and the analgesic effect was greater in more experienced users.[27]

Cannabis may be especially useful for relieving certain specific types of chronic pain. The following account is written by a man suffering from pseudopseudohypoparathyroidism, a hereditary disorder that results from abnormal responses to a hormone secreted by the parathyroid glands. This hormone controls the level of calcium in

25. R. Noyes, Jr., S. F. Brunk, D. A. Baram, and A. Canter, "Analgesic Effect of Delta-9-tetrahydrocannabinol," *Journal of Clinical Pharmacology* 15 (February–March 1975): 139–143.

26. R. Noyes, S. F. Brunk, D. H. Avery, and A. Canter, "The Analgesic Properties of Delta-9-tetrahydrocannabinol and Codeine," *Clinical Pharmacology and Therapeutics* 18 (1975): 84–89.

27. S. L. Milstein, K. MacCannell, G. Karr, and S. Clark, "Marijuana-produced Changes in Pain Tolerance: Experienced and Non-experienced Subjects," *International Pharmacopsychiatry* 10 (1975): 177–182.

the body. When it is deficient or when some of the body's tissues respond to it inadequately (hypoparathyroidism), various symptoms may develop, including muscle spasms, seizures, and, in the variant known as pseudopseudohypoparathyroidism, bone spurs that grow into muscle and nerve tissue and cause agonizing pain.

Irvin Rosenfeld is a thirty-nine-year-old stockbroker from North Lauderhill, Florida. This is his story:

I enjoyed a normal childhood until the age of ten. Then one day, while playing Little League ball, I threw someone out at first and my arm became paralyzed for a short time. The incident upset my parents, so we went to see our family doctor, who took an X-ray of my arm. The X-ray appeared to show a fracture that had healed, leaving jagged bone fragments. It made no sense; I had never broken my arm. The doctor sent us to an orthopedic surgeon, who was equally confused and referred me to Children's Hospital in Boston. After a long series of tests, physicians there concluded that I was suffering from multiple congenital cartilaginous exostosis—a rare disease in which the bones develop buds or spurs that grow out into surrounding muscle and nerve fibers, or inward into the bone itself.

The doctors at Children's Hospital discovered more than 250 bone tumors in my arms, legs, and pelvis. In this disease each tumor can become malignant, but there were so many in my case that they could not all be surgically removed. The rapid, erratic bone growth is intensely painful and may cause crippling injuries. Bone spurs press against nerve bundles, tangle arteries, and prevent smooth muscle functioning. If the spurs are jagged, they rip muscle tissue and lead to internal bleeding. If they erupt suddenly and grow quickly, they can interfere with normal growth and cause crippling deformities. The only saving grace is that multiple congenital cartilaginous exostosis does not last for life. Once you stop growing, around age seventeen, the bone spurs stop forming and growing. In theory, the disease will subside if you don't bleed to death or become permanently crippled in your teens.

To prevent that, I underwent three operations on my left leg and one on my right wrist between the ages of ten and seventeen. But day-to-day problems persisted, mainly because of hemorrhaging and muscle tears. By the age of twelve I was often unable to walk or function normally. I was forced out of public school in the eighth grade and was provided with top-notch tutors by the state of Virginia through graduation. On some days I could walk, even run, but for long periods of time I could barely move. Pain was constant and often unbearable; by age fourteen I needed powerful narcotics to control it. At nineteen I was taking 300 mg a day of Sopor [methaqualone, a powerful sedative] and very high doses of Dilaudid [hydromorphone, an opioid narcotic]. These drugs reduced the pain, but they also diminished my mental acuity and interfered with my life. I did not become addicted, but I became extremely fatigued and at times "out of it." If I cut back in order to be more clearheaded, the pain returned. All I remember, beyond the pain, was the waiting—waiting until I would stop growing.

At seventeen, body scans and X-rays indicated that my tumors had stopped growing. Despite persistent pain, I felt that I had passed the crisis and my condition would soon stabilize. But then, at twenty, another massive bone spur erupted in my right ankle. My doctors assumed that it was a delayed manifestation of a latent growth, and they removed it. They said it would probably be the last tumor I ever had. Instead, it reappeared and grew with amazing speed, until it stretched five inches up my leg and created a bridge of bone that fused my ankle and leg together. Surgery was impossible; the tumor was too large. The doctors decided to amputate my right foot above the ankle.

At this point I questioned my doctors for the first time. It was increasingly clear that my tumors were continuing to grow and new spurs were developing. If I agreed to this, what would need to be amputated next? An arm? Part of another leg? I just said no. No amputation. If the rapidly growing tumor turned malignant, so be it. I was too young to become a cripple for the rest of what might be a short life. I decided to live as well as I could and as whole as I could for as long as I could.

When I was twenty-two, another tumor erupted from my pelvic bone and grew into my groin. This one was surgically removed. Meanwhile, I began to look for other opinions on the nature of my disease. I fruitlessly consulted the Mayo Clinic, the University of Virginia Medical College, the National Institutes of Health (NIH), and the National Cancer Institute (NCI). By this time my drug intake was enormous. I was taking 140 Dilaudid tablets, 30 or more Sopors, and dozens of muscle relaxants and other pills each month. I felt burned out and often walked around in an uncomfortable state. It was difficult to function normally; if I took enough to control the pain, I had difficulty concentrating on my work.

The situation made me dislike drugs intensely. In high school I wrote essays against the use of illegal drugs. It amazed me that people who were well would put a drug into their bodies for fun! I took this attitude with me to college in Florida, where most of the people I met smoked marihuana. At first I strongly resisted "experimenting" with marihuana. I was already "experimenting" with more prescription drugs than my body could handle. But peer pressure works, and I began to smoke marihuana at parties—even though I have never had the slightest idea what people mean when they talk about the high. Perhaps I don't get high because I have spent most of my life taking drugs that are far more powerful than marihuana.

One evening I smoked marihuana with a friend while playing chess. Tumors in the back of my legs made it difficult for me to sit down for more than five or ten minutes at a stretch. But this time I became so absorbed in the game that I remained sitting for over an hour without any pain. I felt I was in one of those "What's wrong with this picture?" ads. When you are conditioned by pain to be in pain and you suddenly aren't in pain, you immediately start asking why. The only unusual thing I had done was smoke marihuana. I never set out to prove to myself that it helped, but after a while it simply became obvious that even a small amount gave me a quality of pain relief I had never before experienced.

I told my doctor, and he suggested that I use marihuana for six months. If I still felt it was helping me after that, we would discuss it again. For the next six months I smoked marihuana regularly. It not only greatly enhanced the quality of pain relief, but drastically decreased my dependence on opioid narcotics and sleeping pills. I became less withdrawn from the world and was able to lead a normal life.

Six months later I reported to my doctor and we discussed the possibility of obtaining marihuana legally. Unfortunately, he died shortly after this conversation and I was forced to begin searching for a new physician. I wrote to an uncle of mine, a pediatrician who lived in Connecticut. He sent me lots of material on marihuana's medical uses, but said he had no idea whether it could be obtained legally.

I had moved back to Portsmouth, Virginia, where I was brought up, and opened a furniture store. This job kept me on my feet moving furniture all day long. I tore muscles and hemorrhaged almost daily. Occasionally these problems would become very serious. When I received the information from my uncle, I took it to the Portsmouth Police Department and explained my medical condition to the chief. I told him I could not afford to buy marihuana on the street and asked permission to smoke marihuana confiscated by the police during raids. The chief said he would look into it. After speaking with a number of people in town— Portsmouth is a small city and my parents are well respected there—he told me that he could not allow me to use confiscated marihuana but would tell the men in his department to leave me alone—as long as I did not sell marihuana but only bought it for medical purposes. There was one other condition—that I never tell anybody about this informal arrangement. I quickly accepted the chief's offer and thanked him.

When I walked into my new doctor's office, he made a number of seemingly trivial observations—the little finger on one hand was unusually large, my arms curved inward, my neck was short, and so on. He then looked at me and said "pseudopseudo-hypoparathyroidism." I wondered if he was all there. He pulled a medical book from a shelf and read me a detailed description of the disease; it matched perfectly, even the relationship with multiple congenital cartilaginous exostosis. The doctor suddenly became very quiet, and I asked him what was wrong. He told me the bone spurs would continue to grow for the rest of my life, and any one of them could become malignant at any time. The resulting cancer would spread quickly and I would die. If cancer didn't get me, a bone spur might pinch my spinal cord and leave me a paraplegic, erupt into a major artery and cause me to bleed to death, or rip into an internal organ and cause permanent, perhaps fatal damage. And the pain would become unbearable.

I asked the doctor if he knew anything about the use of marihuana to control pain and muscle spasticity. He asked me what I knew. I provided him with the information I'd received from my uncle. The doctor promised he would review it, and said he would like to follow my case but did not know how he could legally provide me with marihuana. I liked this doctor very much. Not only was he the first one who actually knew what I had, but he did not reject outright the notion that marihuana might help. He said that if I wanted, I could continue smoking and advise him of any difficulties. It was fairly clear, however, that he doubted marihuana's medical value and assumed I was benefiting from a placebo effect.

For the next few years (1976–1979) I continued to smoke marihuana illegally. Although I did not have to fear arrest, the financial drain was serious; I was spending at least three thousand dollars a year on marihuana. My doctor now agreed to help me if I could find out what needed to be done to get legal approval. One condition was that he never be publicly identified. There was too much craziness surrounding the issue, and he was not willing to risk his career by being identified as a "pot doc." He was outraged that as a licensed physician he could prescribe morphine but not marihuana. It was a maddening situation.

He said he didn't have time to complete a lot of forms, construct elaborate research protocols, or attend to all the administrative demands made by the FDA and other federal agencies that control marihuana. But he was willing to sign on the dotted line if I did the leg work, got the forms filled out, and contacted the proper officials. I had no way of knowing just how hard or how slow it would be. It required many hundreds of phone calls and took not weeks or months, but years.

The law states that the FDA has thirty days to respond to an Investigational New Drug protocol. Forty-five days after sending my doctor's application, we had heard nothing from the FDA, so I called. Officials there politely told me that they had some problems with the IND, but could not say what they were; after all, I was only a patient. They would contact my doctor when they were ready. After another long delay, my doctor called, asked the same question, and received the same vague reply. Several months later, after many additional calls from me, the FDA told my doctor what the problems were. All were minor, mostly insignificant. I sensed that the government was hoping to exhaust my doctor and get him to withdraw his request. The FDA clearly had little interest in the IND and even less in my medical welfare.

Approval finally came nearly a year after the initial request, and the first shipment of legal marihuana did not arrive until several months later. We had to perform elaborate tests to determine what benefits I was receiving; for example, once a week I would go to my doctor's office for an electromyogram (EMG), which measures tension and muscle spasticity. After getting a baseline reading, I would leave the office, go to the parking lot, and smoke one or two marihuana cigarettes. Then I would return and take the EMG again.

I have been legally smoking marihuana (2 percent THC) for four and a half years, ten cigarettes a day. I have had a problem with the law only once, at a business meeting in Florida. I was on my feet all day and didn't get a chance to smoke enough marihuana, so my legs were aching by evening. Dinner was to be held in a hotel banquet room. I've never known how to handle this kind of situation, since I don't want to offend people. But I noticed others around me smoking tobacco, and finally decided I had to smoke, too. My wife suggested that I go to the men's room so that I could have some privacy and avoid bothering anyone. While I was there, a busboy came in, noticed the marihuana smell, and asked me if he could take a couple of "hits" from my cigarette. I refused. He became angry and left.

I realized just how angry he was a few minutes later, when the men's room was raided by the Orlando Vice Squad. The police rushed in and began asking questions. There was a commotion among my business associates as they led me out of the room. I explained that I was using marihuana supplied by the government, legally, for medical purposes. I was told that it didn't matter, since marihuana was illegal under Florida law.

I was placed under arrest and taken to jail. While entering the police station, I tripped on a concrete step, fell, ripped open a blood vessel, and began to hemorrhage. No blood was visible, but my ankle was swelling, and I could not walk. The police officers surrounded me, ordered me to rise, and started pounding their nightsticks into their hands. I began to feel as though I was playing the wrong role in a Grade B movie.

Finally, I managed to convince the officers that I could not get up and needed medical help. A nurse was called. She phoned a doctor, who advised her that it didn't sound too bad. My request to be sent to the hospital was rejected. A wheelchair was provided and I was wheeled in front of a cell. The police confiscated seven pre-rolled NIDA marihuana cigarettes and charged me with possession. Mug shots and fingerprints were taken. I posted bail of $250 and asked for my marihuana cigarettes, but was told they were being kept as evidence. I said fine, I had a tin (about three hundred cigarettes) in my motel room. By this time the police were obviously beginning to fear they had made a mistake, since they did not try to obtain a search warrant.

The arrest occurred on a Friday evening. On Monday morning I managed to reach an FDA attorney who said he would "fix things." A short time later the Florida authorities let me know that they would not prosecute and would expunge the record of my arrest. The police returned my bail money but not my marihuana cigarettes.

From my doctor's annual reports to the FDA and my own experience, I know that marihuana has effectively controlled my pain and allowed me to reduce my use of conventional (and far more dangerous) drugs like Sopor, Dilantin, and Dilaudid. The only problem is that NIDA sometimes fails to meet its commitment and provides marihuana of low potency. When that happens, I am forced to smoke so much that my lungs hurt. Otherwise I have never experienced a serious adverse effect.

The value of marihuana in the treatment of pain and other symptoms following brain surgery is described by Karen Ross in the following account:

In 1988 I had surgery for a malignant brain tumor, an oligodendroglioma. The name is as overwhelming as the reality. Two days after the operation I read an article in the *Boston Globe* about the medical uses of marihuana, especially for people undergoing cancer treatments like radiation and chemotherapy. I had been a moderate user of marihuana before my catastrophic illness, and I took serious note of the article, since I was about to have radiation treatments.

After the surgery I was given dexamethasone, an anti-inflammatory drug, for the swelling in my brain, and Zantac [ranitidine] to protect my stomach from the effects of the dexamethasone.

Within days after returning home I began to have severe anxiety attacks. Sometimes I thought I would lose my mind. I alternately felt as though my chest was going to burst open or be crushed. My hearing was so acute I could hear the bubbles inside a soda can. My speech was slurred, and I mixed up sounds so that people's words sounded like mumbles unless they were talking directly to me. Often I had to rely on lip reading. For these symptoms the doctor gave me Xanax [alprazolam], a tranquilizer, and Elavil [amitryptiline], an antidepressant. The medications helped somewhat, but I was still not comfortable.

My family obtained some marihuana for me and I began to use it along with the Xanax and Elavil. I would smoke at most two "hits" a couple of times a day. I found that marihuana relaxed me and focused my attention, so that I felt less anxiety and rested more easily. It also relieved the pressure in my head better than dexamethasone. I did not experience a "high." I was already in emotional and physical overdrive, and the marihuana put me at cruising speed, regulated and even. Eventually I was able to reduce my use of Xanax and stop using Elavil entirely.

Six weeks after surgery I started taking radiation treatment and went on taking it five days a week for six weeks. Before and after each treatment I smoked marihuana. It allowed me to sleep during the treatment and took away the tightening and tingling sensation I would feel in my head afterward.

The dexamethasone caused me to gain sixty-five pounds. I also developed weakness in my muscles, especially in the knees, insomnia, mood swings, personality changes, potassium loss, and facial hair growth. When the dexamethasone was finally withdrawn, six weeks after the radiation treatments ended, I lost back most of the weight and regained most of my physical strength. My speech also became clearer (I still have a low tolerance for noise and still have to read lips to understand conversations).

All this time I continued to use marihuana. Eventually I returned to part-time work, but shortly afterward marihuana became unavailable. My headache pain, head and eye pressure, facial numbness, anxiety attacks, and slurred speech returned. A brain scan showed no changes in the tumor. When I managed to acquire some marihuana and smoke it, all the symptoms disappeared within a day. A couple of months later marihuana became unavailable again and my symptoms returned like clockwork. This time I was sure why. Friends were able to find some marihuana and put me back on track again. I started to buy a little here and a little there just to be sure I wouldn't get caught short.

I told my primary care physician I was taking marihuana for headache pain, pressure, and slurred speech. He told me he couldn't condone it, especially since it was illegal, but he didn't try to stop me. By now I was able to handle my headaches with regular use of Tylenol, Xanax, and marihuana. On the average a single joint would last me three or four days. On some days I didn't smoke at all.

Ten months later I ran out of marihuana again, and the headaches and anxiety returned. I started taking Tylenol with codeine. I was busy packing to move after twelve years living in my old home, and I thought the stress of moving might have something to do with my problems. I told my oncologist and he suggested a follow-up brain scan, which showed no change.

Afterward, I met with my neurologist. By this time the pain and pressure in my head were becoming more uncomfortable and my speech was more slurred. The neurologist concluded that I was having seizures and prescribed Dilantin [diphenylhydantoin, an anticonvulsant], but it didn't help. I only got worse. It caused insomnia, mental confusion, and decreased coordination. I became frustrated and angry. I called the neurologist and he prescribed dexamethasone again. That didn't help either. He said I had already had the maximum radiation allowable. This kind of tumor does not respond to chemotherapy, and it was doubtful whether further surgery would be effective. My husband and I left his office feeling as though we had two-hundred-pound bricks on our shoulders. Two days later some friends visited and brought some marihuana. I took two hits. Ten minutes later the pressure behind my eye was gone, I had no more headache, the facial numbness had disappeared, and my speech returned to normal.

Four days after seeing the neurologist, my husband and I visited the oncologist again. He said I might be able to have further radiation treatments, since new technology was available, and surgery could always be used as a last resort. Some of that weight we were carrying on our shoulders was lifted. He noticed that my condition had improved, and I told him about the marihuana. He replied, "I am not going to tell you not to do it, and I am not going to tell you to do it, but if it works, as it obviously does, who am I to say differently?"

We left it at that. I decided to stop taking all the prescribed medications—Dilantin, dexamethasone, and Tylenol with codeine—not only because they weren't working but because I was worried about the side effects. Marihuana didn't have any side effects that I noticed.

The morning after I saw my oncologist, I called the neurologist again. He was pleased that my speech had returned to normal and I sounded more upbeat. I told him it had nothing to do with the drugs he had prescribed and I was not going to take them any more. He responded as I expected, saying that he didn't approve, and that marihuana was illegal. He went on, "If that is what your decision is there is nothing I can do to stop you." My husband and I met him again a couple of weeks later and I told the story again. He was very critical and demeaning. He told me that I shouldn't drive and that marihuana is damaging to short-term memory. He acted as though I was sitting around getting high all the time. I tried to explain that I only smoked in the morning or evening or when the symptoms were particularly bad and that there was no "high." I think he was reacting this way because I was in control of my care instead of him.

We have decided to find another doctor who isn't so unyielding, narrow-minded, and pessimistic and, furthermore, is better informed about the new radiation technology. I want to live each

day with hope, happiness, and all the zest life can offer. I know
my problems are far from over and probably never will be, but
I also know I am equipped to manage my life and care, and I
refuse to be treated as though I am not. I will continue to recover
in my own way with the help of marihuana.

The greatest irony in proscribing use of cannabis to relieve pain
is that the best alternatives are addictive and sometimes debilitating opioids. A woman who described her case to us suffers from
melorheostosis, a rare and incurable condition that involves severe
joint pain. When she first developed the disorder, her physician prescribed massive doses of Darvocet, a combination of propoxyphene
(a synthetic opioid) and Tylenol #3 (codeine and acetaminophen).
She needed up to fifteen Darvocets a day to control the pain until she
started to smoke marihuana. She has found that "smoking marihuana
when the pain first starts will round it off. Otherwise it increases very
fast; I begin to feel nauseated and develop cold and hot sweats, simply
from the pain." She could usually control the pain with one to two
joints a day. "But it is a black market item and when we are paying an
average of $75 for a quarter of an ounce and you only have an income
of $444 a month, you don't buy very much. I feel I should not have
to live like a criminal because of the ignorance of politicians. I have
to be terrified about whether police will come and search my home.
Am I going to lose my home and my children because I have found
something that makes me able to cope?"

As a thirty-two-year-old mother of three small children, she found
that cannabis did not compromise her functioning the way large doses
of opioids did: "Marihuana for some reason relaxes my nervous system and allows me to function mentally on a normal basis. When
taking Darvocets and Tylenol I become a different person. I wake
up feeling drugged, I go to sleep feeling drugged, I function like a
drugged person. I lose little bits and pieces of my family because I am
so drugged out that I can't function, even to just sit there and talk to
them or read them a story. As a mother I don't have time to lose with
my children because of a drug-induced state." This woman echoes the

nineteenth-century understanding that cannabis, although it is not as powerful a pain reliever as opioids, has fewer serious side effects and creates no risk of dependence.

MIGRAINE

Migraine is a severe headache that lasts hours to days and is accompanied by visual disturbances or nausea and vomiting or both. The attacks usually are recurrent. They can be brought on in a susceptible person by stress, by certain foods, and by certain types of sensory stimulation (bright light, loud noise, penetrating odors). The onset usually occurs before age twenty and rarely after age fifty. About 20 percent of the population has experienced a migraine attack; women are three times more likely than men to suffer from migraine.

There are several types of migraine. In common migraine, the pain is usually throbbing and often but not always on one side of the head. It is usually accompanied by nausea and vomiting, and it is exacerbated by any movement or noise. In the comparatively rare classical migraine, the attack begins with visual disturbances (including partial blindness and light flashes in the field of vision), and sometimes dizziness, weakness on one side, ringing in the ears, thirst, drowsiness, or a feeling of impending doom. These neurological symptoms are followed by a severe one-sided headache with sensitivity to light and often nausea and vomiting. Classical migraine may also be complicated by tingling, numbness, weakness, or paralysis in various parts of the body. Another type of headache probably related to migraine is the cluster headache, which is more common in men than in women. Here the pain is concentrated around one eye; it is constant rather than throbbing, and it usually wakes the sufferer from sleep. It tends to recur nightly for weeks to months and then disappear for months or even years.

Migraines probably result from dilated blood vessels in the brain. They may begin as a neurological disorder or as a more general failure of metabolic regulation. Levels of the neurotransmitter serotonin have been shown to fall during an attack.

Drugs can be used either to cut short migraine attacks or to prevent long-term recurrence. Chemicals derived from ergot, a fungus that grows on rye, are highly effective in stopping an attack at the early stages; ergot derivatives inhibit the effects of serotonin. Once the headache is fully established, opioids (usually codeine or meperidine) can be used to relieve the pain. Some drugs prescribed for prevention of chronic migraine are methysergide (which is related to the ergot derivatives), beta-blockers, calcium channel blockers, chlorpromazine (Thorazine®), and the steroid prednisone. Ten to 20 percent of sufferers get no relief from these drugs, and many more get incomplete relief or suffer serious side effects.

As we have noted, cannabis was highly regarded as a treatment for migraine in the nineteenth century, yet the topic is almost untouched in the twentieth-century medical literature. Carol Miller, a classic migraine sufferer, describes her experience as follows:

> I first experienced a migraine in a classroom when I was fourteen. The sparkling, flickering visual effects, which were curious at first, consumed me so that I could not see the blackboard. I asked to be excused, let myself into the nurse's room, and vomited for several hours before my mother came to get me.
>
> After this happened several times, my mother took me to see our doctor, a close family friend and neighbor whom I saw very often because I had a lot of allergies. He and my mother agreed that the headaches were caused by the recent death of my baby sister, and he gave me nothing for the nausea and pain. Although headaches continued with some regularity, it wasn't until college that I was given the diagnosis of migraine and received medication. The college infirmary prescribed Ecotrin [coated aspirin], which helped somewhat with the headache but not with the visual effects or the nausea. It also gave me tremendous heartburn.
>
> One time the pain was so severe that they gave me an injection of Demerol [a synthetic opioid], which pretty completely wiped out the pain but left me very lightheaded. At times I took a

banana-flavored syrup [probably codeine] which made me very sleepy. I remember that it was difficult to make it through the final exams because I was so lightheaded, and that my asthma got very bad during this period.

After graduation, while working at Indiana University, I saw a private physician who prescribed Mudrane [a combination drug that includes ephedrine and phenobarbital], which he warned was habit forming. I quit taking them because they seemed to make my blood pressure so low I could hardly work. After moving to San Francisco I was given Darvon [propoxyphene, another opioid], but I took it only briefly because it gave me a rash.

I had been taking aspirin with codeine but found it constipated me terribly. When I became pregnant with my first child, I was very concerned about medication. A friend told me I couldn't take any medication safely and suggested I rely on herbs. I was studying herbal healing and preparing for a natural birth, so this sounded right to me. I tried scullap tea, a light valerian and chamomile tea, and then lavender. The teas were soothing and the slower pace of life after quitting work helped; migraines became rare.

Several years later the migraines returned, and my husband said he had read that marihuana was good for headaches. I was amazed. Two hits and a short rest completely warded off the nausea and headache. As soon as I noticed flickering visuals that forewarned me of an approaching migraine, I could take a little cannabis and a short nap and the migraine would not develop at all. I was usually ready to go back to work in half an hour. It gave me a feeling of tremendous power to be finally in such control of my migraines.

In the eighteen years since I began using cannabis to relieve migraines, I have been caught away from home several times without my herb. Once I tried taking Tylenol and found it helped a little with the pain but not at all with the nausea or the visual effects. Both of my older daughters (now seventeen and twenty-one) also get occasional migraines, which first appeared when they began to menstruate. Both get tremendous relief from cannabis herb. My mother suffers from severe headaches, but she has never used cannabis because it is illegal. She has a horrible time with medications prescribed for her—nausea, constipation, high blood pressure. I often tell her that when marihuana is legal and she uses it for the first time and realizes how she has suffered unnecessarily all these years, she is going to be really furious.

Relief of migraine could be just another analgesic effect of cannabis, but one study suggests that something more is involved. THC has been found to inhibit the release of serotonin from the blood of migraine sufferers during an attack (but not at other times). This result requires confirmation, and its significance remains unclear, but it could be a useful clue to further research.[28]

PRURITIS

Don Spear is a fifty-two-year-old man from Flint, Michigan, who suffers from atopic dermatitis, an inflammatory skin disorder that is probably an allergic reaction of unknown origin. The symptoms are pruritis (severe itching) and patches of inflamed skin, especially on the hands, face, neck, legs, and genitals. It is usually treated with corticosteroids and ointments applied to the skin. Steroids are only partially effective and in any case can be used only occasionally during crises, since long-term use has serious side effects. Antihistamines help to control the itching, but they, too, have limited value. The scratching causes infections that must be treated with antibiotics. Don Spear tells the following story:

I am afflicted with a debilitating, potentially life-threatening skin condition called atopic neurodermatitis. In 1954, as an eighteen-year-old, while stationed at an army base in Texas, I noticed that

28. Z. Volfe, A. Dvilansky, and I. Nathan, "Cannabinoids Block Release of Serotonin from Platelets Induced by Plasma from Migraine Patients," *International Journal of Clinical and Pharmacological Research* 5 (1985): 243–246.

the skin around my eyes was itchy and scaling. At first I thought it was the arid Texas climate, but the condition became worse and spread to other parts of my body. The skin in affected areas became highly irritated, turned dark red, and began to split open. A year later, when the army transferred me to West Germany, much of my body was covered with patches of blistered, bright red skin that would split open, scab, and split open again. These areas became infected from constant scratching.

Doctors in army hospitals in Germany diagnosed my condition as atopic neurodermatitis. I used all the available medications, ointments, and preparations, but nothing helped. My hands and arms were shredded from split, scabbing skin and constant scratching. Gangrene set in, and the doctors considered amputating both my arms at the elbow. In a last effort to prevent amputation, my forearms were completely bandaged so that I could not scratch them; I was also given massive doses of antibiotics and the new "wonder drug," cortisone. For the itching, which nearly drove me out of my mind, the doctors prescribed tranquilizers and sedatives. My arms were saved, but I could not tolerate any more cortisone. Despite the army's best efforts, my skin condition could not be controlled. In January 1956, I was discharged with a 50 percent service-connected disability.

In the next ten years I tried nearly every available prescription and over-the-counter drug: heavy doses of Librium, Valium, and other addictive tranquilizers, cortisone creams and ointments, coal-tar baths and preparations. None provided long-term relief. I was hospitalized several times because of infections that resulted from uncontrollable itching and split skin.

Because my skin condition was disfiguring, it was difficult to find work. Employers would not hire me and other workers did not want to work with me. I finally took a job with the Fisher Body Company, but I repeatedly needed prolonged sick leave. After ten years the company computed that I had taken six years of sick leave and retired me. Looking for work to support my wife and four children, I again discovered that many people simply would not hire me. The skin disease persisted. I would often wake up at night and find that blood had oozed from my scalp onto the pillow. The itching was so severe and intense that I used sandpaper on my skin to get relief. My marriage broke up, and I became very withdrawn and frightened.

In the spring of 1973, a friend of mine who had served in Vietnam told me that he smoked marihuana there and found it enjoyable. I was reluctant, not only because it was illegal but also because I did not like to use drugs of any kind. I had long since given up alcohol and tobacco, and my experience with prescription drugs made me even more cautious. I come from a strict, moral background in which drug use is not regarded as right.

Finally, one weekend at a drag race, I took a few puffs from my friend's marihuana cigarette. I may also have taken a couple of puffs from another cigarette the next day. I noticed nothing unusual after smoking, no mental effects. On Tuesday or Wednesday of the following week I realized that a particularly bad area of skin looked much less red and inflamed. It occurred to me that the itching had not been bothering me for several days. I wondered whether marihuana had anything to do with the unexpected improvement, but did not give the idea much credit.

The next weekend my friend and I went to another drag race, and he offered me marihuana again. By this time the itching had returned, but it stopped suddenly with the first puff. I was astonished. After years of using every drug and skin product available without gaining relief, the itching stopped with one puff of a marihuana cigarette. For the next three years I continued to smoke marihuana only on weekends, and never more than a few puffs at a time. My skin condition improved dramatically. Because I was no longer scratching, the split skin healed. Then the red patches began to fade and were replaced by normal skin. Soon I was no longer disfigured. I got a regular job and became a solid worker. I no longer had to take sick leave.

In early 1977 my older brothers discovered that I was smoking marihuana and told our parents. Although I was over forty, I cared very deeply for their feelings. I explained the situation to them, but I could see they were not convinced. They feared that I had become addicted. I told them I would stop smoking marihuana for three months and see what happened. I had never experienced any adverse mental or physical effects, and I had no difficulty quitting. I developed no craving and had no "shakes" or "sweats." But within three days my entire body was itching. The skin between my toes and fingers became irritated and inflamed. The inflammation quickly spread up my hands and feet to my arms and legs, then to my scalp, head, and chest. Within weeks my skin was splitting, I was scratching constantly, and dark red welts appeared over much of my body. I was becoming disfigured again, and there was blood on the sheets at night. My parents and brother became alarmed and pleaded with me to start smoking marihuana again. I was reluctant, because I did not like to be called an addict. Finally, I realized that my family did not care whether marihuana was illegal. They only cared about its effect on my skin.

I began smoking on weekends again. This time it took nearly a year before my skin was back to normal. I continued to smoke marihuana for the next decade, until February 1987, and my skin condition remained under control. I maintained a good employment record, and never smoked while working. In February 1987, I learned that my company intended to conduct random urinalysis tests on its employees. I requested help from my union representatives, and meanwhile asked doctors at the Veterans' Administration to help me obtain marihuana legally. They referred me to the V.A. Drug Rehabilitation Unit, where I was told that I did not have a drug problem. In effect, the doctors there decided that I was simply using the drug therapeutically. They encouraged me to continue smoking marihuana. But the threat of urine testing and possible loss of my job deeply upset me. Confused, not knowing what to do, I stopped smoking. My skin condition almost immediately erupted.

After a few weeks it was serious and rapidly growing worse.

My parents, my brother, good friends, and even my union representative encouraged me to start smoking marihuana again. The alternative was to obey the law and live with a deforming skin condition that might, through infection, kill me. I took sick leave and started to grow my own marihuana.

In December 1989 a neighbor told the police. I was arrested and convicted. The punishment was a large fine, house arrest for four months, and two years of probation. The judge said that all charges would be dropped if I obtained a legal prescription. But I have had to stop smoking because of the urine tests at work. Since I stopped again (December 1989), the itching has been almost constant, and my skin repeatedly splits open and leaks fluid on my feet, hands, scalp, legs, chest, and even penis.

Marihuana is the only drug that prevents both the skin lesions and the horrible itching. If marihuana were legal, I could control this hell of a disease. Marihuana might also help thousands of people with similar skin problems, but there is no research because it is a prohibited drug and doctors do not like political controversy.

MENSTRUAL CRAMPS AND LABOR PAIN

Two common uses of cannabis in the nineteenth century were for the treatment of menstrual cramps and reduction of labor pains. Although there is no twentieth-century medical literature on the topic, many women have experimented with cannabis, and for some it is the drug of choice, especially in the relief of menstrual cramps. The following account illustrates both uses, as well as relief of nausea in pregnancy:

> I am a thirty-seven-year-old housewife. I run a small business, volunteer in my daughters' school and chaperone class trips. I appear to be "straight" and many of my neighbors and acquaintances have no idea I smoke marihuana. I have had painful menstrual cramps for many years. In 1976 a laparoscopy revealed

ovarian cysts and endometriosis. I was told that the endometriosis would return after an operation, so I decided not to have one. I had hormone shots for several months, but stopped because I was afraid of cancer. Prescription painkillers made me feel too drugged to function efficiently as a mother. At that time I used pot as a recreational drug, smoking it socially with friends, and I accidentally found out that it also relieved my menstrual cramps. Now most of my friends don't even know I smoke, but I light up as soon as my menstrual period starts.

I had my first baby in 1972, when I was only seventeen. The doctors gave me a shot to put me to sleep and when I woke up I had a very lethargic baby. We spent three days in the hospital. In 1979, when I had my second baby, I went to natural childbirth classes and later smoked pot on the way to the hospital. It greatly relaxed me and thus relieved some of the pain, but the effect lasted only about an hour and a half. I was in the hospital for only twenty hours this time, and I was amazed at how much more alert and hungry the second baby was compared to my first poor drugged baby.

In 1991 I became pregnant again. In my seventh month, I became nauseated, had heartburn, and began to vomit two to four times a day—so much I wasn't gaining weight. The doctor decided the cause was pressure from the baby on the valve at the top of my stomach. I began smoking pot before meals, and after that I vomited only twice a week. The baby weighed nine pounds at birth. I wonder how small she would have been if I hadn't used my favorite antinausea drug.

This time when I had the baby I stayed home and smoked pot for the first seven hours of labor. I delivered less than three hours after arriving at the hospital, and the pain was no problem until the pot wore off, just before I delivered. This time I was not surprised that the baby was alert and hungry. We went home six hours after birth; I spent less than nine hours at the hospital, and wasn't even billed for a whole day.

DEPRESSION AND OTHER MOOD DISORDERS

For most people, depression is a passing mood; for some, it is a debilitating chronic illness with severe physical as well as emotional symptoms. When it is deep and persistent enough to interfere with work, friendships, family life, or even physical health, depression is regarded as a psychiatric disorder—one of the most common and one of the most serious.

An episode of severe, or major, depression may last several weeks to several years. One set of symptoms is inconsolable misery accompanied by despair and guilt. Victims feel worthless and inadequate; they have no hope for the future and ruminate about death and suicide. They may think that they have lost all their money or are being punished for grave sins or dying of incurable diseases. Some depressed persons do not admit sadness or guilt; instead, they withdraw from human contacts, lose all interest in life, and become incapable of feeling pleasure. Time passes slowly for them and the world seems dreary and meaningless. Normal emotional responses, even ordinary despondency or grief, become impossible. They are fretful and irritable. They cannot concentrate or make even minor decisions. They turn the same few ideas over and over in their minds. Some depressed patients are listless and lethargic, with slow movements, toneless speech, and an expressionless face—in extreme cases, muteness and immobility resembling catatonic stupor. Others pace, weep, moan, and wring their hands in anxious agitation. In bipolar or manic-depressive disorder, major depression alternates with uncontrollable elation, or mania.

Depression is not simply a disorder of mood. Depressed people lack energy in every sense, physical as well as emotional and intellectual. The dominant symptoms may be loss of appetite and insomnia (or, sometimes, oversleeping and a ravenous appetite), backaches, headaches, upset stomachs, constipation, and above all chronic fatigue. People who claim to be "tired all the time" may be depressed even if they acknowledge no sadness or despair. Manic persons, on the other hand, are sleepless and tireless—until they become exhausted and break down.

The standard treatments for depression are the many antidepressant drugs introduced in the past forty years. These drugs are effective for a wide range of symptoms, including not only various mood disorders but also what would once have been diagnosed as personality disorders. The most popular class of antidepressants is the tricyclics, including imipramine (Tofranil®), amitryptiline (Elavil®), desipramine (Norpramin®), and several other drugs. Their most common side effects are dry mouth and blurred vision. Others are weight gain, constipation, difficulty in urinating, and orthostatic or postural hypotension (dizziness caused by a reduced blood flow to the brain on sitting up or standing up). They can be risky for patients with cardiovascular disease, since they increase the heart rate and may disturb cardiac rhythm.

Another group of antidepressants is the monoamine oxidase (MAO) inhibitors: isocarboxazid (Marplan®), tranylcypromine (Parnate®), and phenelzine (Nardil®). They may cause dizziness, insomnia, and impotence and when used in combination with such foods as red wines, pickles, and certain cheeses, which contain the substance tyramine, can produce dangerously high blood pressure. Because of these potentially serious side effects, they are rarely a first choice in treating depression, but they may be helpful for patients who do not improve on other drugs.

About a third of depressed patients do not respond to tricyclics or MAO inhibitors or cannot tolerate their side effects. Some of these patients can be treated with one of the newer antidepressants introduced in the last few years, the most popular of which is fluoxetine (Prozac®). Its side effects include occasional nausea, weight loss, and agitation (or, in some patients, drowsiness).

The preferred treatment for both mania and depression in bipolar disorder is lithium carbonate. It, too, is only partially effective, and its many side effects include weight gain, hand tremors, drowsiness, excessive thirst or urination, and potential damage to the heart, kidneys, and thyroid gland. Patients often stop taking lithium either because of these side effects or because it takes some of the joy from their lives along with the manic episodes. It has been described as a "loose-fitting emotional strait jacket."

Cannabis first appeared in the Western medical literature as a suggested treatment for depression in the mid-nineteenth century. In 1845, Jacques-Joseph Moreau de Tours proposed its use in melancholia (especially with obsessive rumination) and chronic mental illness in general.[29] In the next hundred years a number of medical papers supported and disputed the utility of cannabis in the treatment of various mental illnesses. In 1947, in an uncontrolled study, G. T. Stockings, an English physician, administered a synthetic cannabinoid to fifty depressed patients, and thirty-six showed definite improvement. Obsessive ruminations were significantly reduced in six out of seven patients.[30] In 1948, D. A. Pond tried unsuccessfully to replicate these results.[31] A double-blind study involving fifty-seven patients suffering from severe melancholia or milder depression was conducted in 1950 by C. S. Parker and F. W. Wrigley; they found no difference between the synthetic cannabinoid and a placebo. But they used a smaller dose than Stockings had used (10–20 mg as opposed to 15–90 mg), saying it was necessary to do so because the drug had such a strong sedative effect.[32] Synthetic cannabinoids with less sedative activity may yet prove to be useful in treating depression.

The most recent study on cannabis and depression was undertaken in 1973. Eight hospitalized patients were given either THC or a placebo for up to a week. The THC did not relieve their depression, and in four of the patients it produced discomfort and anxiety so serious

29. J.-J. Moreau de Tours, "Lypemanie avec stupeur; tendance a la demence.—traitement par l'extrait (principe resineux) de cannabis indica—Guerison," *Lancette Gazette Hôpital* 30 (1857): 391.

30. G. T. Stockings, "A New Euphoriant for Depressive Mental States," *British Medical Journal* 1 (1947): 918–922.

31. D. A. Pond, "Psychological Effects in Depressive Patients of the Marihuana Homologue Synhexyl," *Journal of Neurological and Neurosurgical Psychiatry* 11 (1948): 279.

32. C. S. Parker and F. W. Wrigley, "Synthetic Cannabis Preparations in Psychiatry: I Synhexyl," *Journal of Mental Science* 99 (1950): 276–279.

it had to be withdrawn. The authors questioned whether "different effects might be observed in other settings or in patients with less severe depressive symptoms." They also noted that "the administration of THC under double-blind conditions in this trial precluded the establishment of any positive expectations in the patient. The fact that the patients could not have prepared themselves for the experience of an altered state of consciousness may also have contributed to the predominantly negative effects of the drug in these depressed patients. Finally, the relatively brief duration of the trial (one week) must be kept in mind since standard antidepressants require two to three weeks to produce clinical improvement."[33]

Today, among the minority of depressed patients who do not respond to any of the standard antidepressants or find the side effects unbearable, some have discovered that cannabis is more useful than any legal drug. We first learned about the following patient's use of cannabis from her psychiatrist. She called us because she was puzzled to find that marihuana was more useful than the drugs she had prescribed, and she wished to be reassured of its safety. The patient gives her account below:

> I am a thirty-nine-year-old health professional who suffers from chronic depression. I have been able to graduate from college, receive a postgraduate degree with highest honors, and establish a successful professional career, but it has been a constant struggle. No matter how much I accomplished, how much praise I received, none of it registered. I could only ruminate about my shortcomings, and I seemed to have no control over my unrealistic negative thoughts.
>
> My first major episode of depression occurred in 1969, when I went away to college. I withdrew halfway through my freshman year and began semi-weekly therapy sessions with a psychiatrist. With her help and the use of a tricyclic antidepressant, I was able to return to a college closer to home the following September. I

33. J. Kotin, R. M. Post, and F. K. Goodwin, "Delta-9-tetrahydrocannabinol in Depressed Patients," *Archives of General Psychiatry* 28 (1973): 345–348.

continued to see her once a week until I left the East in August of 1976. While at school in the Midwest, I saw a psychiatrist renowned for his expertise in the pharmacological treatment of depression. Since I returned to the East in 1981, I have been in therapy once again with my original psychiatrist, either once a week or every two weeks.

Under the guidance of these therapists I have tried more than a dozen different drugs, including several types of tricyclic antidepressants, Prozac, lithium, Ritalin [methylphenidate, a stimulant related to amphetamine], synthetic thyroid hormone, and probably others I have forgotten. The only ones that have affected my moods significantly are Elavil at high doses and combinations of Dexedrine [dextroamphetamine] and a barbiturate. Elavil works only during an incapacitating episode of depression, and its side effects, especially constipation, are distressing. Since use of Dexedrine and barbiturates as antidepressants is considered unorthodox, my therapist and I have been uneasy about it, but it was the only medication that worked. Several prominent psychiatrists have verified this and recommended that I use whatever helps. But now I am becoming tolerant to both of these drugs (I have been careful not to increase the dose, because I know the dangers).

In the spring of 1990 I smoked marihuana for the first time since 1973. To my amazement, a quarter of a joint changed my self-perception to match the person others saw. It was like night and day. I had experienced a similar change only a few times before, when Elavil kicked in and lifted me out of the depths. But with Elavil it took four days of rapidly increasing doses; with marihuana it took less than five minutes, every time. Since then I have been using marihuana to think clearly, to concentrate, and simply to enjoy the beauty of the world in a way I couldn't for years.

I try to carry the same positive feelings with me while I am not directly under the influence of marihuana. I now use marihuana as an antidepressant once or at most twice a day. No one realizes

I am smoking it, because I don't act stoned. I have been cutting back on my other medications and often forget to take them. After smoking some cannabis in the morning, I no longer dread the responsibility of going to work but actually look forward to it. I have always awakened in the morning more exhausted than when I went to sleep. Even during weekends and vacations, I have found it difficult to get dressed and get moving. Immediately after I smoke marihuana, all that changes. I feel energetic and loquacious; I want to socialize, exercise, or do whatever needs to be done. I feel a passion for life. I even see myself differently in the mirror, and realize that I am not the homely beast I usually see. While using marihuana I realized that I was not spending time with the person I wanted to be with, so I ended an unsatisfying relationship of two and a half years. I am now with someone I love dearly. Without marihuana I have an orgasm only through masturbation or after heroic efforts during intercourse. Cannabis transforms me into a fully developed sexual human being. I can easily shut out inappropriate thoughts and enjoy what I am feeling. I can have orgasms by stimulation practically anywhere on my body, even just through kissing—amazing!

It is unfair and cruel that the antidepressant that helps me most (and is probably, in its pure form, least toxic) is unavailable for legal prescription. I have to break the law to obtain it and pay exorbitant prices for a drug whose cost of production is minimal.

Another patient who suffers from episodic depression writes as follows:

I am a forty-seven-year-old white male, a partner in a multi-million dollar company. . . . As soon as I started school my emotional problems became apparent, and an endless trek to various health professionals began. My school phobia made me sneak away from school, sometimes by climbing out windows. I spent much time being interviewed by "special ed" teachers and social workers. From early on I was examined by a continuous flow of physicians. My earliest recollection is the one who prescribed special arches for my shoes (to relieve headaches) and a syrup at night to make me sleep.

The headaches persisted; the depressions became paralyzing episodes that occurred several times a year and lasted days to weeks. Because of them I missed much of grade school and junior high.

In my sophomore year of high school, things got worse. I was given a prescription for Miltown [meprobamate, an anti-anxiety drug]. I took it in varying dosages for several months. It caused me to become drowsy and dizzy; my speech slurred, and I developed chronic diarrhea. My poor performance in school worsened. I started to lose my coordination. My depressions continued, perhaps made worse. I was glad to stop using it.

My experience with Miltown was so unpleasant that I refused to take any other "mental" drugs for the next two years. I did see a therapist on a weekly basis. His diagnosis was "episodes of acute depression."

During this period I managed to just barely complete high school, and got accepted at a small local college. During my second semester I attempted suicide. I was told by a doctor that I had an "obsessive-compulsive personality." It was suggested that I take Librium. I started taking this drug and found myself in a continuing state of depression, confusion, and lethargy. I had to leave school. When my speech started slurring, I abandoned the Librium.

I got a job driving a truck, and started seeing a new doctor, a psychiatrist. After nine months I reapplied to college and was accepted. The doctor convinced me to try another drug, Tofranil, that he said was very effective in treating depression. I started using it and soon found I was losing all power of concentration. I became restless, full of anxiety. It became almost impossible to urinate. I developed a lump the size of a marble in my left nipple. The doctor ascribed these symptoms to the Tofranil. I stopped using it and again left school. My depression was still there, and I was desperate for some relief. I also started getting pains in my stomach. A GI series revealed a duodenal ulcer. I constantly chewed antacids and took tablets called Zantac.

Life was becoming more difficult, and the doctor suggested another medicine, Vivactil [protryptiline, a tricyclic antidepressant]. Again, the side effects were disastrous. I became more agitated than before, had great trouble urinating, and a chronic skin disease I have (atopic dermatitis) started to itch with a fury. I developed a peculiar taste in my mouth that would not leave and had a continual feeling of nausea. Shortly after discontinuing Vivactil I was in the psychiatric ward of a New York hospital, suffering from "atypical depression."

In the hospital I was put on lithium. After two days my hands started to shake. This tremor became so intense that after one week I was unable to write or hold a glass without spilling the contents. I had diarrhea and nausea; my vision started to blur.

I ceased using the lithium and left the hospital after a stay of two weeks. When I saw my therapist again, he made an unusual statement: "I'm not suggesting this," he said, "if I did I could lose my license, but have you ever tried marihuana?" I had smoked something alleged to be marihuana once in high school and had been unaffected. I thought it might be worth another try. I called a friend I suspected would know where or how to obtain some, and the next day she brought me two joints. I later learned that her husband (who is a dentist) used marihuana to ease the pain of chronic depression.

Remembering my previous experience, I had low expectations. Alone in my room I lit the first joint. Soon I found myself lost in reverie. Previously, when I was depressed, the sadness became the focal point of my existence. Now my mind was being distracted by neutral, and even funny or pleasant thoughts. The constant pain of the depression was reduced to an occasional nagging ache. I slept well and awoke feeling refreshed, not "doped up" and lethargic. It soon became apparent that when I was in the throes of a depressive episode, a marihuana cigarette was a greater source of relief than anything I had ever tried before—not a cure, but something that diluted the pain. The marihuana permitted me to function better than any licit drug. I didn't become drowsy, develop tremors, or have any of the side effects associated with the drugs I had previously taken. I gained an appetite I never had, and put needed weight on an emaciated frame. I found myself having ideas that would not ordinarily have come to me, some practical, some not. I was able to pierce the black cloud that surrounded me and climb out far enough to meet my responsibilities. The use of marihuana makes it impossible for depressive thoughts to become the total focus of my life.

The fact that marihuana is illegal made me search for a licit medicine that was at least as effective. The next one I was given was Norpramin. This chemical offered no relief and came with an assortment of side effects that aggravated my prostate, gave me diarrhea, left a terrible, lingering taste in my mouth, and colored my tongue black. For about a year I was given Adapin [doxepin, another tricyclic] with only minor side effects, but it did little or nothing to change my condition. I was also given Buspar [buspirone, an anti-anxiety drug], which seems to have no effect at all. Perhaps the very worst of them all was Prozac, which actually made me more anxious, nauseous, dizzy to the point of fainting, and unable to achieve orgasm. I have also had Desyrel [trazodone], which causes only minor side effects, but again seems to do little good.

As of this writing, I have smoked marihuana for more than two decades. In addition to dampening the pain of depression, I have found it reduces nausea and burning in the stomach due to the production of acid. It allows me to sleep peacefully. It stimulates my imagination when working on creative projects. It enhances simple joys, such as eating M&Ms or walking in the woods. Since its use jeopardizes my freedom, I would prefer a legal substitute. So far I have found none.

I use no other illicit substances. I do not use tobacco. My alcohol intake is no more than an occasional drink on a Saturday night out. I usually have one cup of tea a day and two glasses of Coca-Cola. I take several aspirins a week.

The following account was written by a forty-one-year-old woman with apparent manic-depressive disorder.

I was born on Friday, October 13, 1950, a few months before my father had his first serious bout with manic depression. My mother said he was taking valuable art objects they owned and throwing them down the trash chute in their New York apartment building.

I enjoyed my youth with a great deal of abandon. How much of this would be mood disorder I could not tell you. As a single person I didn't notice; I just rode the waves of emotional highs and lows and didn't think much about it. I was an old pro at this by the time I was nineteen and met my husband. It was only through my association with him that I came to terms with my mood problems, although right before I met him I had checked myself in at a mental health clinic complaining that I sometimes felt unable to concentrate on one thing at a time.

I think I was twenty-two years old when my troubles cropped up again. At one point my husband and I went to see a psychologist. We talked about my mood swings and spells of nervousness, anger, and depression. The tiniest negative thing happening would cause long-lasting rage, very hard to quell. We told the psychologist of my father's history, even longer and grislier by then. He must have been in every state mental institution along the East coast. My grandmother, his mother, was wasting away by this time, losing her lifelong battle with chronic depression. I don't know much about her case except that she was chronically sad and starved herself to death after her husband passed away.

This man said my husband and I needed to lose weight; that was the extent of his advice. We did not see him much longer. By this time I was experiencing most of the symptoms I have today, although they have strengthened year by year. Sometimes I feel elated, exhilarated, with a great deal of energy. It sounds great, but you can get to be feeling so good that you scare the people around you, believe me! This is accompanied by light sleeping and nocturnal habits. I tend to become angry or aggressive when it is not appropriate, or just talk too loud. I often have a low self-image or feel sad. I sometimes have a hard time getting up to work, a heaviness that keeps me from moving. I get racing thoughts that make concentration hard. I have strong emotions that change rapidly. I tend to be physically clumsy. I develop unexplained skin rashes, and sometimes feel like I'm generating electricity and shooting it out my fingers and toes. My judgment is often poor.

It was in my early twenties that I first used the herb cannabis for my condition. I had been exposed to it several times, the first when I was quite young. My mother had taken me to a mental health center after my initial signs of trouble as a child. After a group therapy session there some of the other kids took me riding and gave me a joint. Nothing at all happened, and I concluded it must be a mild drug.

When I was exposed to it later, I would actually choose it over alcohol because it didn't have such strong and negative effects on me. This is how I discovered that it was effective against most of my symptoms. Suppose I am in a fit of manic rage—the most destructive behavior of all. A few puffs of this herb and I can be calm. My husband and I have both noticed this; it is quite dramatic. One minute out of control in a mad rage over a meaningless detail, seemingly in need of a strait jacket, and somewhere, deep in my mind, asking myself why this is happening and why I can't get a handle on my own emotions. Then, within a few minutes, the time it takes to smoke a few pinches—why, I could even, after a round of apologies, laugh at myself!

But this herb is illegal and I have a strong desire to abide by the law. My father was having great success with a new drug, lithium carbonate. I saw my father's physician and he recommended that I try it. I took lithium for six months and experienced several adverse side effects—shaking, skin rashes, and loss of control over my speech. But I would still be taking it if it had worked for me as it did for my father. It literally restored his life. I had gotten worse, if anything.

The combination of lithium side effects and increased manic-depressive symptoms drove me back to the use of cannabis. Some years later I tried to go without it again, this time because of increased social pressure against illegal drug use. It was a very difficult time for my family. Whenever I started to become manic, my husband and son would get scared and cower, triggering rage and making matters worse. When depression struck it was a black funk on our household. And I can tell you from the experience with my father, this can really destroy a family. After a while the knowledge that a little bit of herb would help me so much became irresistible. At first I tried eating cannabis, but soon returned to smoking because I could control the dose better.

The legal situation now is worse than ever. I jeopardize my freedom and property in order to control my condition. Do I have a choice? I don't at all consider myself a drug abuser. I am doing what any rational person in my position would do. Cannabis does not cure my condition and over the years it has probably continued to worsen. But with judicious use of this medicine my life is fine. I can control things with this drug that seems so harmless compared to the others I've tried, including tranquilizers as well as lithium. I am constantly concerned that I will be cut off from my supply of marihuana or caught with it in my possession. I feel my sanity may depend on it. Cannabis lessens what is troubling me and returns me to a more normal state. Often I do not experience a "high" at all, just a return to normal.

OTHER MEDICAL USES

Cannabis also has some more speculative potential medical uses:

Asthma

About ten million Americans suffer from asthma—attacks of breathlessness and wheezing caused by the narrowing of small airways in the lungs, the bronchioles. The linings of the bronchioles become inflamed and swollen and fill with phlegm; a chronic cough may develop from attempts to free the obstruction. Asthma attacks kill more than four thousand Americans each year. The disorder is caused by allergic reactions to pollen, dust, feathers, and animal hair, as well as by cold air, infections, exercise, and air pollutants. It is more common in children than adults and usually grows less severe with age. Bronchodilators can be used to relax the bronchial muscles and widen the airway; synthetic steroids reduce inflammation and the resulting swelling. But beta-agonists, the drugs most commonly used as bronchodilators, may cause sleeplessness, jitteriness, and nausea; and steroids, used for more than a few months, have more serious side effects, including bone loss, seizures, and bleeding. (These can be mitigated somewhat if an inhaler is used to deliver the steroid directly to the lungs, bypassing the bloodstream). Other anti-inflammatory drugs also have serious side effects and are more difficult to administer.

Given the limitations of existing drugs in the treatment of asthma, use of cannabinoids should be considered. Several studies have shown that THC acts as a bronchodilator in both normal subjects and patients with either chronic bronchial asthma or experimentally induced bronchial spasms. In one study, THC allowed a freer flow of air in and out of the lungs of healthy subjects; in asthmatic patients, it reversed bronchial constriction. In a related study, smoked THC was compared with inhaled isoproternol, a standard bronchodilator. Both drugs relieved bronchial spasms; isoproternol worked faster and had a stronger peak effect, but the effect of THC lasted longer.[34] Whole

34. D. P. Tashkin, B. J. Shapiro, and I. A. Frank, "Acute Pulmonary Physiologic Effects of Smoked Marihuana and Oral Delta-9-tetrahydrocannabinol in Healthy Young Men," *New England Journal of Medicine* 289 (1973): 336–341; D. P. Tashkin, B. J. Shapiro, Y. E. Lee, and C. E. Harper, "Effects of Smoked Marihuana in Experimentally Induced Asthma," *American Review of Respiratory Disease* 112 (1975): 377–386.

marihuana is probably not useful for this purpose, because the irritating effects of THC and the tars in marihuana smoke have the potential to produce chronic bronchitis in heavy users. Cannabis smoke also contains carcinogens and substances that are toxic to the cilia, hairlike cells that help free the lungs of mucus.

The alternatives to smoking are oral use and spray inhalers. But the antiasthmatic activity of oral THC is delayed and unreliable because of its erratic absorption. When THC is delivered as an aerosol spray, some experiments have found significant dilation of the bronchi without adverse effects. In one experiment, THC in aerosol form produced a faster but shorter-acting effect than the standard bronchodilator isoproternol.[35] This line of research has not been pursued because THC in spray form is still a bronchial irritant.[36] Nevertheless, there are compelling reasons to continue research. Other cannabinoids, natural or synthetic, may prove to be more effective than THC or have fewer side effects. Safer ways of delivering these drugs may be discovered. Finally, the mechanism of action of cannabinoids is apparently different from that of other bronchodilators, and new treatments may be developed if that mechanism can be identified. The need for new approaches is indicated by a recent article demonstrating that the use of beta-agonist bronchodilators is riskier than previously believed and is associated with high death rates in asthma sufferers.[37]

Insomnia

Cannabis has a long history as a hypnotic (sleep-inducing) drug, and many people use it for that purpose today, including one of the multiple sclerosis patients who tells her story above. There is now ex-

35. L. Vachon, A. Robins, and E. A. Gaensler, "Airways Response to Aerosolized Delta-9-tetrahydrocannabinol: Preliminary Report," in *The Therapeutic Potential of Marijuana,* ed. S. Cohen and R. C. Stillman (New York: Plenum, 1976).

36. D. P. Tashkin, S. Reiss, B. J. Shapiro, B. Calverese, J. L. Olson, and J. W. Lodge, "Bronchial Effects of Aerosolized Delta-9-THC in Healthy and Asthmatic Subjects," *American Review of Respiratory Disease* 115 (1977): 57–65.

37. W. O. Spitzer, S. Suissa, P. Ernst, et al., "The Use of Beta-agonists and the Risk of Death and Near Death from Asthma," *New England Journal of Medicine* 326 (1992): 501–506.

perimental evidence that the hypnotic effects are produced by canna-bidiol rather than THC. One controlled study of fifteen insomniacs found that over a five-week period "sleep quality was significantly influenced by 160 mg of cannabidiol as two-thirds of the subjects slept more than seven hours. . . . Most subjects had few interruptions of sleep and reported having a good night's sleep."[38] Legally available hypnotics leave much to be desired. Tolerance develops to most of them, many cause rebound insomnia, some are addictive, and all have the potential for a lethal overdose. Given these drawbacks, it is unfortunate that the hypnotic potential of cannabis in general and of cannabidiol in particular has not been more thoroughly explored.

Other Causes of Severe Nausea

Cancer and AIDS patients are not the only ones who can make use of marihuana's antinauseant and appetite-stimulating effects. It has also been used by women who suffer from the rare disorder known as hyperemesis gravidarum—a greatly heightened form of morning sickness in which the sufferer is never free of nausea and vomiting throughout pregnancy. In the past, abortion was sometimes necessary to save the woman's life. More recently these women have been hospitalized and fed intravenously. Some have now discovered that they can do without intravenous feeding by smoking marihuana daily. Although it is preferable for pregnant women not to use drugs, cannabis probably poses less risk to the fetus than prolonged intra-venous feeding or standard antiemetic drugs.

Kidney failure is another potential cause of severe nausea. The following account was written by James C. Longcope, M.D., a psychiatrist:

> George Duborg was hospitalized in September 1991 with all the symptoms of major depression. He slept in two-hour snatches. He lacked appetite and energy, and had lost fifty to sixty pounds in two months. He was irritable and his concentration was poor.

38. E. A. Carlini and J. M. Cunha, "Hypnotic and Antiepileptic Effects of Canna-bidiol," *Journal of Clinical Pharmacology* 21 (1981): 417S–427S.

He had not been able to distract himself by reading for several weeks, and although he was a baseball fan, he could not even muster any interest in the World Series. Although he was not suicidal, he said he wished "someone would put me out of my misery."

At age sixty-two, George was a successful investment broker with a stable marriage and healthy children, all of them out of college and making their way in the world. But he had a lot to be depressed about, since he had lost the function of his kidneys. Several months before the hospitalization he had taken a nonsteroidal anti-inflammatory agent for intractable migraine headaches. It caused partial kidney failure, which became total kidney failure after an idiosyncratic reaction to an intravenous diagnostic procedure. He was being sustained by renal dialysis as he waited for a kidney donor.

But George's problem was not just renal failure or depression. It was a symptom that had become more devastating than his disease: nausea. Spasms of nausea and hiccoughs waxed and waned but never went away. The dialysis was adjusted and minor electrolyte imbalances were corrected, but the nausea persisted. Compazine did not help. Zantac did not help. Zofran, a widely heralded new intravenous antinausea drug, did not help, even when given every two hours. The antidepressant nortriptyline had to be discontinued because of liver toxicity. When I introduced myself, George said, "I don't need a psychiatrist. I need something for this terrible nausea. I will deal with my depression and my fate, if you give me a level playing field."

His internist had ordered Marinol (tetrahydrocannabinol) and the hospital pharmacy was trying to obtain it. Although he was willing to try anything, we decided to wait for the Marinol. On October 19 it arrived and George received three 5 mg doses in the next twenty-four hours. On October 20 I stopped by to see how he was doing. "See, I told you," he said, "give me a level playing field and I will manage my fate." He was playing gin with his wife and invited me to join. "We would be glad to have your company until the World Series comes on; just don't pull any psychiatrist tricks. I am doing fine; this stuff works. I can barely remember how bad I was." It was like finding Sam Magee "sitting cool and calm in the heart of the furnace roar." George needed Marinol again on the next three days, and then went twenty-four hours without it. The nausea and hiccoughs came and went several times over the next few weeks, and each time 5–10 mg of Marinol controlled the symptoms.

Today George is alive and well. Because his kidney function spontaneously recovered, he was able to discontinue dialysis. Even the migraine headaches have improved, or at least don't seem quite as bad. Tetrahydrocannabinol had helped him through the worst phase when nothing else worked.

If the reports and studies we have been discussing are correct, marihuana in its natural form might have been just as effective or even more so.

Antimicrobial Effects

Another possible medical use of cannabis is suggested by the work of some investigators at Palacky University in Olomouc, Czechoslovakia. They found that cannabis extracts containing cannabidiolic acid produce impressive antibacterial effects on a number of microorganisms, including strains of staphylococcus that resist penicillin and other antibiotics. They successfully treated a variety of conditions, including ear infections, with cannabis lotions and ointments. Topical application of cannabis relieved pain and prevented infection in second-degree burns. The Czech researchers report that a pathologist injured his thumb in the dissecting room and the resulting infection resisted all available treatments. Amputation was being considered when a cannabis extract overcame the infection. If these findings are confirmed, they may prove especially important at a time when so many bacterial strains have become resistant to available antibiotics.[39]

Cannabis may also be useful for the symptomatic relief of a viral

39. J. Kabelik, Z. Krejci, and F. Santavy, "Cannabis as a Medicament," *Bulletin of Narcotics* 12 (1960): 20–22; Z. Krejci, "On the Problem of Substances with Antibacterial Action: Cannabis Effect," *Casopis Lekaru Ceskych* 43 (1961): 1351–1354.

disease, herpes. People who suffer cold sores or genital herpes have steeped marihuana in rubbing alcohol until the solution turns greenish and dabbed it on the site of an imminent herpetic sore outbreak. They say it prevents blistering and makes the sores disappear in a day or two. So far these reports are only anecdotal, but they are certainly worth following up. There is now some evidence that THC actually binds to the herpes virus and inactivates it.[40]

Antitumoral Effects

The relief of nausea and vomiting in chemotherapy is not the only proposed use of cannabis in cancer treatment. In the 1970s an experiment was conducted in which the lungs of mice were injected with cancer cells and delta-9-THC, delta-8-THC, or cannabinol was applied; the size of the tumors dropped 25 to 82 percent, depending on dose and duration of treatment, with a corresponding increase in survival time.[41] Other animal studies also suggest that some cannabinoids have tumor-reducing properties. Although there is no human and little other research in this field, cannabinoids may prove to be useful as adjuncts to other chemotherapeutic agents.

Dystonias

In 1981 it was reported that patients with idiopathic dystonia improved when they smoked marihuana. This is a group of disorders characterized by abnormal movements and postures resulting from prolonged spasms or muscle contractions.[42] Animal studies confirmed

40. G. Lancz, S. Specter, H. K. Brown, J. F. Hackney, and H. Friedman, "Interaction of Delta-9-tetrahydrocannabinol with Herpes Viruses and Cultural Conditions Associated with Drug-induced Anti-cellular Effects," in *Drugs of Abuse, Immunity, and Immunodeficiency*, ed. H. Friedman et al. (New York: Plenum, 1991), 287–304; G. Lancz, S. Specter, and H. K. Brown, "Suppressive Effect of Delta-9-tetrahydrocannabinol on Herpes Simplex Virus Infectivity in Vitro," *Proceedings of the Society for Experimental Biology and Medicine* 196 (1991): 401–404.

41. L. S. Harris, A. E. Munson, and R. A. Carchman, "Antitumor Properties of Cannabinoids," in *The Pharmacology of Marihuana*, ed. M. C. Braude and S. Szara, 2 vols. (New York: Raven, 1976), 2:773–776.

42. C. D. Marsden, "Treatment of Torsion Dystonia," in *Disorders of Movement: Current Status of Modern Therapy*, vol. 8, ed. A. Barbeau (Philadelphia: J. B. Lippincott, 1981), 81–104.

that cannabinoids might have antidystonic properties, and another human experiment was undertaken in 1986. Cannabidiol was given, along with standard medications, to five patients with dystonic movement disorders. A dose-related improvement ranging from 20 to 50 percent was observed in all patients over a six-week period. Side effects were minimal.[43] As far as we know, this potential medical use of cannabis has not been explored further. Dystonias are often produced by the neuroleptic drugs given to patients with chronic psychotic disorders. The symptoms can be disfiguring and incapacitating, and present treatments are inadequate. Psychiatrists who must prescribe antipsychotic drugs might consider exploring the use of cannabidiol to counter this serious side effect.

IN DEFENSE OF ANECDOTAL EVIDENCE

It is often objected, especially by federal authorities, that the medical usefulness of marihuana has not been demonstrated by controlled studies. We have already discussed the several controlled experiments with large numbers of subjects suggesting an advantage for marihuana over oral THC and other medicines. But controlled studies have their limitations. They can be misleading because the wrong patients are studied or the wrong doses used. The focus of such studies is a statistically significant effect on a group, but medicine has always been concerned with the needs of individual patients. Idiosyncratic therapeutic responses to a drug can be obscured in group experiments. In these experiments there is often little effort to identify the features of patients that affect drug responses.

Physicians also have available evidence of a different kind whose value is often underestimated. It commands much less attention than it once did, yet it is the source of much of our knowledge of synthetic medicines as well as plant derivatives. As Louis Lasagna, M.D., has pointed out, controlled experiments were not needed to recognize the

43. P. Consroe, R. Sandyk, and S. R. Snider, "Open Label Evaluation of Cannabidiol in Dystonic Movement Disorders," *International Journal of Neuroscience* 30 (1982): 277–282.

therapeutic potential of chloral hydrate, barbiturates, aspirin, curare, insulin, or penicillin. He asks why regulators are now willing to accept the experiences of physicians and patients as evidence of adverse effects but not as evidence of therapeutic effects.[44]

There are many more recent examples of the value of anecdotal evidence. It was in this way that the use of propranolol for angina and hypertension, of diazepam for status epilepticus, and of imipramine for childhood enuresis was discovered, although these drugs had been originally approved by regulators for other purposes. A famous recent example is minoxidil, which was developed by the Upjohn Company to lower blood pressure. The company had no idea that topical application could restore lost scalp hair. But anecdotal evidence (later confirmed by controlled studies) was so persuasive that the company now markets it mainly as a treatment for baldness. Another drug, tretinoin (Retin-A®) was originally marketed as an acne treatment. Anecdotal evidence that it had antiwrinkle properties led to formal studies proving its effectiveness for that purpose. Further studies have now been inspired by new anecdotal evidence that it can erase liver spots—brownish freckle-like blemishes on the hands and face of older people caused by exposure to sunlight.

As early as 1976 several small and methodologically imperfect studies, not widely familiar in the medical community, had shown that taking an aspirin a day could prevent a second heart attack. Then, in 1988, a large-scale experiment demonstrated effects so dramatic that the researchers decided to stop the experiment to publish the lifesaving results. On one estimate, as many as twenty thousand deaths a year might have been prevented from the mid-1970s to the late-1980s if the medical establishment had been quicker to recognize the value of aspirin. The lesson is suggestive: marihuana, like aspirin, is a substance known to be unusually safe and with enormous potential medical benefits. There is one contrast, however; it was impossible to be sure about the effect of aspirin on heart attacks without a long-

44. L. Lasagna, "Clinical Trials in the Natural Environment," in *Drugs between Research and Regulations,* ed. C. Stiechele, W. Abshagen, and J. Koch-Weser (Darmstadt: Steinfopff Verlag, 1985), 45–49.

term study involving large numbers of patients, but the above reports show that cannabis often brings immediate relief of suffering, measurable in a study with only one subject. Anecdotes or case histories of the kind narrated in this book are, in a sense, the smallest research studies of all.

In the experimental method known as the single-patient randomized trial, active and placebo treatments are administered randomly in alternation or succession to a patient. The method is often useful when large-scale controlled studies are impossible or inappropriate because the disorder is rare, the patient is atypical, or the response to the treatment is idiosyncratic.[45] Donald Spear, Greg Paufler, and Robert Randall, three of the patients who tell their stories in this book, carried out a somewhat similar experiment on themselves when they alternated periods of cannabis use with periods of no use. In Paufler's case the target symptom was muscle spasms, in Spear's, itching, and in Randall's, loss of vision. Admittedly, cannabis was not administered randomly in alternation with a placebo, but the psychoactive effects of marihuana are usually unmistakable, and few patients or observers would be deceived by a placebo. This kind of experiment, of course, has limitations. It can be used only for disorders that are stable and chronic, and the effect of the treatment must be both fairly rapid and fairly quickly reversible on discontinuation. Nevertheless, it is certain that cannabis won its reputation as a medicine partly because many other patients around the world carried out the same kind of experiment.

Anecdotes present a problem that has always haunted medicine: the anecdotal fallacy or the fallacy of enumeration of favorable circumstances. If many people suffering from, say, muscle spasms caused by multiple sclerosis take cannabis and only a few get much better relief than they could get from conventional drugs, those patients would stand out and come to our attention. They and their physicians would

45. E. B. Larson, "N-of-1 Clinical Trials: A Technique for Improving Medical Therapeutics," *Western Journal of Medicine* 152 (January 1990): 52–56; G. H. Guyatt, J. L. Keller, R. Jaeschke, et al., "The N-of-1 Randomized Controlled Trial: Clinical Usefulness," *Annals of Internal Medicine* 112 (1990): 293–299.

understandably be enthusiastic about cannabis and might proselytize for it. These people are not dishonest, but they are not dispassionate observers. Therefore, some may regard it as irresponsible to suggest on the basis of anecdotes that cannabis may help people with a variety of disorders. That might be a problem if cannabis were a dangerous drug. But we believe it is not irresponsible to share these stories for the simple reason that, as we shall see, cannabis is so remarkably safe. It may not work for everyone, but it is most unlikely to do any harm. If the relevant large-scale studies were to be conducted, we might learn that cannabis helps a very large percentage of patients with multiple sclerosis and other disorders. But even in the unlikely event that only a few people get the kind of relief described in this book, it could be argued that cannabis should be available for them because it costs so little and the risks are so small.

3 Weighing the Risks

The benefits of any medicine must be weighed against the risks. Fortunately, there is unusually good evidence on the potential health hazards of marihuana—far better than the evidence on most prescription drugs. Not only has cannabis been used for thousands of years by many millions of people, but there is much recent research inspired by the federal government's interest in discovering toxic effects to justify its policy of prohibition. The potential dangers of marihuana when taken for pleasure and its possible usefulness as a medicine are historically and practically interrelated issues: historically, because the arguments used to justify suppression of recreational use have had a disastrous influence on views of its medical potential; practically, because it is more likely to be safe as a medicine if it is relatively safe as an intoxicant. As the evidence makes it increasingly clear that cannabis is relatively benign, it is becoming harder and harder to deny that a risk-benefit analysis satisfies all requirements for medical use.

Toxic effects of a drug can be classified as either acute (resulting from a single dose) or chronic (resulting from long-term use); a distinction can also be made between physical and psychological (or behavioral) effects.

Table 1   Toxicity of THC, Barbiturates, and Alcohol

	Effective Dose	Lethal Dose	Safety Factor
Secobarbital	100–300 mg	1,000–5,000 mg	3–50
Alcohol	0.05–0.1%	0.4–0.5%	4–10
Tetrahydro-cannabinol	50 mcg/kg	2,160,000 mcg/kg*	40,000*

*Because no human fatalities have been documented, the figures given are for the human effective dose and the lethal dose for mice.

Source: T. H. Mikuriya, "Historical Aspects of *Cannabis sativa* in Western Medicine," *New Physician* (1969): 905.

ACUTE EFFECTS

The most common acute physical effects of smoking or ingesting cannabis or THC are a slight conjunctival hyperemia (reddening of the eyes) and a slightly increased heart rate. Neither of these is uncomfortable or dangerous. After five thousand years of cannabis use by hundreds of millions of people throughout the world, there is no credible evidence that this drug has ever caused a single death. The lethality of drugs is ordinarily measured by a value called the LD50, the dose that will cause 50 percent of animals or human beings taking it to die. The LD50 for cannabis in human beings is not known, because there are no data from which it can be derived. The toxicity of a drug can be estimated by a number known as the therapeutic ratio or safety factor, defined as the lethal dose divided by the effective dose. The toxicity of THC in comparison with barbiturates and alcohol is indicated in table 1. The safety factor for secobarbital (Seconal®) is 3–50 and for alcohol it is just 4–10. The safety factor for THC, as extrapolated from data in mice, is 40,000. Many cancer chemotherapy drugs have a safety factor of 1.5 or even less. Marihuana in its natural form is possibly the safest therapeutically active substance known to humanity.

Marihuana does have some acute behavioral or psychological effects that are of concern. Attention and short-term memory, tracking, and coordination can be impaired under its influence. There is uncertainty about whether these effects persist for some time after the feeling of intoxication has passed.[1] Cannabis shares this drawback with other psychoactive drugs used as medicines, such as the benzodiazepines (including Valium®, Xanax®, and Halcion®). When doctors prescribe these medicines, they caution patients against driving and tell them they may feel slightly sedated at work. Cannabis requires similar cautions. A patient who is given 10 mg of diazepam (Valium®) for sedation before a minor outpatient surgical procedure is forbidden to leave the hospital for some hours, and then only when accompanied. People who use cannabis before cancer chemotherapy might be treated similarly.

Opinions differ on the danger of driving or operating other machinery under the influence of cannabis. Data are scarce and can be interpreted in different ways. Thus, one authority states: "Clearly, marijuana is a substance which produces serious behavioral toxicological effects. Any situation in which safety, both for self and others, depends upon alertness and capability and control of man-machine interaction precludes the use of marijuana."[2] Another group of researchers comes to a different conclusion:

> Several investigators have reported that marijuana reduces risk-taking propensity and driving speed. Because of these compensating tendencies, it is presently not possible to assess the net impact of marijuana as a causal agent in traffic accidents. Although some increased risk appears likely, the magnitude of the risk remains obscure. . . . Many of the laboratory studies which have shown the greatest psychomotor impairment have utilized tasks

1. L. D. Chait, "Subjective and Behavioral Effects of Marijuana the Morning after Smoking," *Psychopharmacology* 100 (1990): 328–333; J. A. Yesavage, V. O. Leirer, M. Denari, and L. E. Hollister, "Carry-over Effects of Marijuana Intoxication on Aircraft Pilot Performance: A Preliminary Report," *American Journal of Psychiatry* 142 (1985): 1325–1329.
2. H. Moskowitz, "Marihuana and Driving," *Accident Analysis and Prevention* 17:4 (1985): 323–345.

that are only abstractly related to driving. . . . it does not necessarily follow that performance on a highly novel and complex laboratory test designed to magnify performance decrements is correlated with actual "real world" performance in a vehicle. The fact that attempts to measure response to simulated accident situations have not consistently detected a marijuana-induced decrement, even at high doses, underscores the need for much research.[3]

If marihuana users try to compensate for impairment by speeding less and generally taking fewer risks, alcohol, by contrast, induces recklessness.[4] On the other hand, one study of 1,023 trauma patients found that 35 percent of all accident victims had THC in their blood, and 34 percent had alcohol (17 percent had both drugs).[5] This survey included all kinds of accidents, not just those involving automobiles. The results, as presented, suggest that although alcohol plays a disproportionate role in automobile accidents caused by recklessness and speeding, marihuana may present greater hazards where attention and forgetfulness are more important. The authors of this study do not take into account that THC found in the blood after an accident is not necessarily a sign of cannabis intoxication, since it may remain in the body for days or even weeks after the last use of cannabis. Nevertheless, persons who fly airplanes, drive trains, and operate heavy machinery under the influence of any psychoactive drug may present a threat, and cannabis is no exception. Accidents are probably its foremost health hazard. Complex tasks requiring rapid decisions, especially in the operation of machinery, are most sensitive to its effects; people who ignore this fact may be jeopardizing themselves and others.

3. R. C. Peck, A. Biasotti, P. N. Boland, C. Mallory, and V. Reeve, "The Effects of Marijuana and Alcohol on Actual Driving Performance," *Alcohol, Drugs, and Driving: Abstracts and Reviews* 2:3–4 (1986): 135–154.

4. G. B. Chesher, "The Effects of Alcohol and Marijuana in Combination: A Review," *Alcohol, Drugs, and Driving: Abstracts and Reviews* 2:3–4 (1986): 105–120.

5. C. A. Soderstrom, A. L. Trifillis, B. S. Shankar, et al., "Marijuana and Alcohol Use among 1023 Trauma Patients: A Prospective Study," *Archives of Surgery* 123 (June 1988): 733–737.

Two other acute "side effects" of medical cannabis must be considered. By far the most common of these is the high, or altered state of consciousness. As described by recreational users, this state lasts two to four hours when cannabis is smoked and five to twelve hours when cannabis is taken by mouth. Its most common form is a calm, mildly euphoric state in which time slows and sensitivity to sights, sounds, and touch is enhanced. The smoker may feel exhilarated or hilarious. Thoughts flow rapidly and short-term memory is reduced. Body image and visual perception undergo subtle changes. Often it is as though the cannabis-intoxicated adult perceives the world with some of the wonder and curiosity of a child; details ordinarily overlooked capture the attention, colors seem brighter and richer, and new values may appear in works of art that previously seemed to have little or no meaning. Sometimes drowsiness or sleep ensues after an hour or two.

As several authors above indicate, not everyone experiences this effect, and some, like Stephen Jay Gould, dislike it, but most regard it as pleasurable and interesting. Marihuana not only relieves their symptoms but makes them feel better generally. In the words of a fifteen-year-old boy receiving chemotherapy whose demoralizing nausea and vomiting was prevented by marihuana, "Pot turns bad things into good." We must caution the reader that this experience is exquisitely sensitive to conditions of psychological "set" (expectations and mood) and social setting. In particular, descriptions of recreational use cannot necessarily be extrapolated to a medical setting.

The other, much less common but still significant acute psychological effect of marihuana is a state of anxiety, sometimes accompanied by paranoid thoughts and occasionally mounting to a temporarily incapacitating panic. The condition is self-limiting, and simple reassurance is the best treatment. Perhaps the main danger to the user is being diagnosed as psychotic. There are no hallucinations, and the capacity to test the reality of thoughts and perceptions—the sine qua non of sanity—remains intact.

Anxiety and paranoid thoughts are most likely to occur in an inexperienced user taking the drug in an unpleasant or unfamiliar setting. These reactions become less common as familiarity with the drug grows. It has been noted repeatedly by government commissions studying marihuana that sophisticated users know when they have had enough and are able to titrate the dose to prevent themselves from becoming too highly intoxicated. In a recent study demonstrating this capacity, experienced marihuana smokers were given cigarettes containing 0.0, 1.3, or 2.7 percent THC. When the dose was higher, they took shorter puffs and inhaled less smoke.[6]

Obviously the danger of an anxiety or paranoid reaction is magnified when the drug is illegal, its potency is unknown or uncertain, and the patient is alone and without guidance. The reaction should be easy to avoid in a comfortable medical setting where physicians can determine the dose and prepare patients for the psychoactive effects. When cannabis is a legal medicine, patients will suffer anxiety reactions even more rarely than they do now.

Cannabis is also sometimes said to cause an acute psychosis, described as a prolonged reaction with symptoms that include delusions, hallucinations, inappropriate emotions, and disordered thinking. The reaction is rarely reported in the United States, and given the many millions of marihuana smokers in this country, the evidence for it would be less equivocal if it occurred with any regularity. Most reports of cannabis psychosis come from India and North Africa. An authority often cited is A. Benabud of Morocco, but his description of the symptoms is far from clear; they seem to resemble other acute toxic states, including, especially in Morocco, those associated with malnutrition and endemic infections. Benabud estimates the number of kif (marihuana) smokers in Morocco suffering from psychosis as not more than five in a thousand.[7] But this is lower than the rate of all psychoses in the populations of other countries. If Benabud's estimate is correct, we would have to conclude that, if anything, marihuana protects smokers against psychosis.

---

6. S. J. Heishman, M. L. Stitzer, and J. E. Yingling, "Effects of Tetrahydrocannabinol Content on Marijuana Smoking Behavior, Subjective Reports, and Performance," *Pharmacology, Biochemistry and Behavior* 34 (February 1989): 173–179.

7. A. Benabud, "Psychopathological Aspects of the Cannabis Situation in Morocco: Statistical Data for 1956," *Bulletin of Narcotics* 9 (1957): 2.

A report by the American psychiatrist Walter Bromberg lists thirty-one psychoses attributed to marihuana. Of these thirty-one cases, however, seven involved patients already predisposed to psychoses that were only precipitated by the drug, seven others were later found to be schizophrenic, and one was later diagnosed as manic-depressive.[8] In a study examining 1,238 cannabis users in India, 13, or 1 percent, were found to be psychotic; this is the average rate of chronic schizophrenia in the total population of Western countries.[9] In a study conducted by the LaGuardia Commission, nine of seventy-seven persons had a history of psychosis, but they were all patients in hospitals or other institutions. Allentuck and Bowman, the psychiatrists who examined this group, concluded that "marihuana will not produce psychosis de novo in a well-integrated, stable person."[10]

An article by V. R. Thacore and S. R. P. Shukla in 1976 revived the concept of the cannabis psychosis.[11] The authors compared twenty-five cases of what they call a paranoid psychosis precipitated by cannabis with an equal number of paranoid schizophrenics. The cannabis psychotics are described as patients who had developed a psychosis after prolonged abuse of cannabis. All had used cannabis heavily for at least three years, mainly in the form of bhang, the weakest of the preparations common in India. In comparison with the schizophrenic patients, the cannabis psychotics are described as more panicky, elated, boisterous, and communicative; their behavior is said to be more often violent and bizarre, and they are said to have flight of ideas without schizophrenic thought disorder. The prognosis is said to be good; the symptoms are relieved by phenothiazines, and recurrence is prevented by avoiding cannabis.

8. W. Bromberg, "Marihuana Intoxication: A Clinical Study of *Cannabis sativa* Intoxication," *American Journal of Psychiatry* 91 (1934): 303.

9. H. B. M. Murphy, "The Cannabis Habit: A Review of the Recent Psychiatric Literature," *Addictions* 13 (1966): 3.

10. S. Allentuck and K. M. Bowman, "The Psychiatric Aspects of Marihuana Intoxication," *American Journal of Psychiatry* 99 (1942): 248.

11. V. R. Thacore and S. R. P. Shukla, "Cannabis Psychosis and Paranoid Schizophrenia," *Archives of General Psychiatry* 33 (1976): 383–386.

Thacore and Shukla did not provide enough information to justify the view that all these conditions were either a single clinical syndrome or related to cannabis use. They said little about the actual amount used, except that relatives regard it as abnormally large; they did not discuss why the psychosis was associated with bhang rather than the stronger cannabis preparations. The meaning of "prolonged abuse on more than two occasions" in the case of men who are constant heavy cannabis users was not clarified, and the temporal relation between the cannabis use and the psychosis was not specified. The cannabis-taking habits of the control group of schizophrenic patients were not discussed. It seems likely that the patients described as cannabis psychotics had a variety of syndromes, including acute schizophrenic reactions, acute manic episodes, severe borderline conditions, and a few symptoms actually related to acute cannabis intoxication—mainly anxiety reactions and a few psychoses of the kind that may arise in unstable people under any stress or after any change in consciousness or body image.

In fact, our own clinical experience and that of others[12] suggests that cannabis may exacerbate psychotic tendencies in some schizophrenic patients when the illness is otherwise reasonably well controlled with antipsychotic drugs. Even in these patients, it is often difficult to tell whether the use of cannabis is precipitating the psychosis or merely an attempt at self-treatment for the early symptoms (needless to say, the two possibilities are not mutually exclusive).[13]

12. D. A. Treffert, "Marihuana Use in Schizophrenia: A Clear Hazard," *American Journal of Psychiatry* 135 (1978): 10.

13. It is interesting to note that recent research suggests that cannabidiol has some antipsychotic activity. Rats given the drug apomorphine develop stereotyped sniffing and biting behavior. Drugs with known antipsychotic activity in human beings suppress this behavior; in one experiment, researchers have found that cannabidiol also suppresses it. Another characteristic correlated with antipsychotic activity is a tendency to increased secretion of the hormone prolactin, which is also produced by cannabidiol. Some researchers have even suggested that cannabidiol belongs to the same group as the atypical antipsychotic drugs, including the highly effective clozapine. A. W. Zuardi, J. Antunes Rodrigues, and J. M. Cunha, "Effects of Cannabidiol in Animal Models Predictive of Antipsychotic Activity," *Psychopharmacology* 104 (1991): 260–264.

There is no reason to believe that cannabis causes or contributes to the onset of schizophrenia itself.[14]

Like many other drugs, cannabis can produce a toxic delirium when taken at very high doses, especially by mouth. The symptoms are confusion, agitation, disorientation, loss of coordination, and sometimes hallucinations. This is not a cannabis psychosis; the delirium persists only as long as large amounts of the drug are present in the brain. Unlike the delirium caused by many other drugs, it is not associated with serious physiological changes and is not physically dangerous.

One rather rare reaction to cannabis is the flashback, or spontaneous recurrence of drug symptoms while not intoxicated. Although several reports suggest that flashbacks may occur in marihuana users even without prior use of any other drug,[15] in general they seem to occur only in those who have previously used psychedelic drugs. There are also some people who have flashback experiences of psychedelic drug trips while smoking marihuana; this is sometimes regarded as an extreme version of a more general heightening of the marihuana high that occurs after the use of hallucinogens. Many people find flashbacks enjoyable, but to others they are distressing. They usually fade with the passage of time.

CHRONIC EFFECTS

In some medical uses of cannabis—for example, the relief of nausea during cancer chemotherapy—there is no need to be concerned about long-term effects. But patients who use cannabis regularly for long periods of time, as in the treatment of glaucoma, may smoke as many as ten cigarettes a day, every day. In these cases we must consider possible chronic toxic effects, both physical and psychological (or behavioral). As a result of federal government efforts

14. G. Thornicroft, "Cannabis and Psychosis: Is There Epidemiological Evidence for an Association?" *British Journal of Psychiatry* 157 (1990): 25–33.

15. V. P. Ganz and F. Volkman, "Adverse Reactions to Marijuana Use among College Students," *Journal of the American College Health Association* 25 (1976): 93.

to demonstrate the harmfulness of recreational use, there is now a vast literature on this topic. Although a study can be found to support almost any view, the findings are on the whole strikingly reassuring.

One of the first questions asked about any psychoactive drug is whether it is addictive or produces dependence. This question is hard to answer because the terms *addiction* and *dependence* have no agreed-upon definitions. Two recognized signs of addiction are tolerance and withdrawal symptoms; these are rarely a serious problem for marihuana users. In the early stages, they actually become more sensitive to the desired effects. After continued heavy use, tolerance to both physiological and psychological effects develops, although it seems to vary considerably among individuals. Almost no one reports an urgent need to increase the dose to recapture the original sensation. What is called behavioral tolerance is probably a matter of learning to compensate for the effects of the high. It may explain why farm workers in some third world countries are able to perform heavy physical labor while smoking a great deal of marihuana and why glaucoma patients who smoke ten times a day can go about their lives without apparent interference from the drug. Behavioral tolerance substantially reduces the effects of intoxication on attention and motor coordination in long-term users.

A mild withdrawal reaction has been reported in experimental animals and apparently in some human beings who take high doses for a long time. The symptoms are anxiety, insomnia, tremors, and chills lasting for a day or two. It is unclear how common this reaction is; in a Jamaican study, even heavy ganja users did not report abstinence symptoms when they were deliberately withdrawn from the drug during an experiment.[16] None of the patients who tell their stories in this book experienced withdrawal symptoms when they had to stop using cannabis because they feared the law or lacked money to purchase the drug. To the extent that a withdrawal reaction exists, it clearly does not present serious problems to marihuana users or cause them to go on taking the drug.

16. V. Rubin and L. Comitas, *Ganja in Jamaica* (The Hague: Mouton, 1975).

In a more important sense, dependence means an unhealthy and often unwanted preoccupation with a drug to the exclusion of most other things. People suffering from psychological dependence on a drug find that they are constantly thinking about it, using it, or recovering from its effects. The habit impairs their mental and physical health and hurts their work, family life, and friendships. They often know that they are using too much and repeatedly make unsuccessful attempts to cut down or stop. These problems seem to afflict proportionately fewer marihuana smokers than users of alcohol, tobacco, heroin, cocaine, or even benzodiazepines, such as diazepam (Valium®). Even heavy users in places like Jamaica and Costa Rica do not seem to be dependent in this damaging sense.

It is often difficult to distinguish between drug use as a cause of problems and drug use as an effect; this is especially true in the case of marihuana. Most people who develop a dependency on marihuana would also be likely to develop other dependencies because of anxiety, depression, or feelings of inadequacy. The original condition is likely to matter more than the attempt to relieve it by means of the drug.

Much attention has also been devoted to the so-called stepping-stone hypothesis—the theory that marihuana smoking leads to the use of opiates and other dangerous drugs. In this country, almost everyone who uses any other illicit drug has smoked marihuana first, just as almost everyone who smokes marihuana has drunk alcohol first. Anyone who uses any given drug is more likely to be interested in others, for some of the same reasons. People who use illicit drugs, in particular, are somewhat more likely to find themselves in company where other illicit drugs are available. None of this proves that using one drug leads to or causes the use of another. Most marihuana smokers do not use heroin or cocaine, just as most alcohol drinkers do not use marihuana. The metaphor of a stepping-stone suggests that if no one smoked marihuana it would be more difficult for anyone to develop an interest in opiates or cocaine. There is no convincing evidence for or against this. What is clear is that at many times and places marihuana has been used without these drugs, and vice versa.

Apart from the issue of dependence and the stepping-stone theory, the idea has persisted that in the long run marihuana smoking causes some sort of physical or mental deterioration. It would not be unreasonable to suppose that long-term use of the more potent forms of cannabis might have debilitating effects, as prolonged heavy drinking does. But the evidence is weak. One of the earliest and most extensive investigations of this question was conducted by the British government in India in the 1890s. The investigating agency, called the Indian Hemp Drugs Commission, interviewed some eight hundred persons—including cannabis users and dealers, physicians, superintendents of insane asylums, religious leaders, and a variety of other authorities—and in 1894 published a report of more than three thousand pages. In it, the commission concluded that there was no evidence that moderate use of the cannabis drugs produced any disease or mental or moral damage or that it tended to lead to excess any more than the moderate use of whiskey.[17]

In the LaGuardia study in New York City, an examination of chronic users who had averaged seven marihuana cigarettes a day for eight years showed no mental or physical decline.[18] Several later controlled studies of chronic heavy use have failed to establish any pharmacologically induced harm.[19] A more recent government-sponsored review of cannabis conducted by the Institute of Medicine also found little evidence of its alleged harmfulness.[20]

17. *Report of the Indian Hemp Drugs Commission, 1893–1894,* 7 vols. (Simla: Government Central Printing Office, 1894); D. Solomon, ed., *The Marihuana Papers* (Indianapolis: Bobbs-Merrill, 1966).

18. Mayor's Committee on Marihuana, *The Marihuana Problem in the City of New York* (Lancaster, Pa.: Jacques Cattell, 1944).

19. M. H. Beaubrun and F. Knight, "Psychiatric Assessment of Thirty Chronic Users of Cannabis and Thirty Matched Controls," *American Journal of Psychiatry* 130 (1973): 309; M. C. Braude and S. Szara, eds., *The Pharmacology of Marihuana,* 2 vols. (New York: Raven, 1976); R. L. Dornbush, A. M. Freedman, and M. Fink, eds., "Chronic Cannabis Use," in *Annals of New York Academy of Sciences* 282 (1976); J. S. Hochman and N. Q. Brill, "Chronic Marihuana Use and Psychosocial Adaptation," *American Journal of Psychiatry* 130 (1973): 132; Rubin and Comitas, *Ganja in Jamaica.*

20. Institute of Medicine, *Marijuana and Health* (Washington, D.C.: National Academy, 1982).

These conclusions are confirmed by three major studies conducted in Jamaica, Costa Rica, and Greece. In these studies researchers compared heavy long-term cannabis users with nonusers and found no evidence of intellectual or neurological damage, no changes in personality, and no loss of the will to work or participate in society.[21] The Costa Rican study showed no difference between heavy users (seven or more marihuana cigarettes a day) and lighter users (six or fewer cigarettes a day). Studies in the United States find no effects of fairly heavy marihuana use on learning, perception, or motivation over periods as long as a year.[22]

On the other side are clinical reports of a personality change called the amotivational syndrome. Its symptoms are said to be passivity, aimlessness, sloth, apathy, uncommunicativeness, and lack of ambition. Some proposed explanations are hormone changes, brain damage, sedation, or depression induced by marihuana. Since the amotivational syndrome does not seem to occur in Greek or Caribbean farm laborers, some writers suggest that it affects only skilled and educated people who need to do more complex thinking.[23]

The problem of distinguishing causes from symptoms is particularly acute here. Some cannabis users in India and the Middle East may be hungry, sick, or hopeless and trying to soften the impact of

---

21. Rubin and Comitas, *Ganja in Jamaica*; W. E. Carter, ed., *Cannabis in Costa Rica: A Study of Chronic Marihuana Use* (Philadelphia: Institute for the Study of Human Issues, 1980); C. Stefanis, J. Boulougouris, and A. Liakos, "Clinical and Psychophysiological Effects of Cannabis in Long-term Users," in *Pharmacology of Marihuana*, ed. Braude and Szara, 2:659–666; P. Satz, J. M. Fletcher, and L. S. Sutker, "Neurophysiologic, Intellectual, and Personality Correlates of Chronic Marihuana Use in Native Costa Ricans," in *Annals of the New York Academy of Sciences* 282 (1976): 266–306.

22. C. M. Culver and F. W. King, "Neurophysiological Assessment of Undergraduate Marihuana and LSD Users," *Archives of General Psychiatry* 31 (1974): 707–711; P. J. Lessin and S. Thomas, "Assessment of the Chronic Effects of Marihuana on Motivation and the Achievement: A Preliminary Report," in *Pharmacology of Marihuana*, ed. Braude and Szara, 2:681–684.

23. W. Carter and P. Doughty, "Social and Cultural Aspects of Cannabis Use in Costa Rica," *Annals of the New York Academy of Sciences* 282 (1976): 1–16; Rubin and Comitas, *Ganja in Jamaica*; C. Stefanis, R. Dornbush, and M. Fiuk, *Hashish: Studies of Long-term Use* (New York: Raven, 1977).

an unbearable reality. Heavy drug users in our own society are often bored, depressed, and listless or alienated, cynical, and rebellious. Sometimes the drug causes these states of mind, and sometimes they result from personality characteristics that lead to drug abuse. Drug abuse can be an excuse for failure or a form of self-medication. Because of these complications and the absence of confirmation from controlled studies, the existence of an amotivational syndrome caused by cannabis use must be regarded as unproven.

Much recent research on the health hazards of marihuana concerns its long-term effects on the body. Studies have examined the brain, the immune system, the reproductive system, and the lungs. Suggestions of long-term damage come almost exclusively from animal experiments and other laboratory work. Observations of long-term marihuana users in the Caribbean, Greek, and other studies reveal little disease or organic pathology associated with the drug.[24] For example, there are several reports of damaged brain cells and changes in brain-wave readings in monkeys smoking marihuana, but neurological and neuropsychological tests in Greece, Jamaica, and Costa Rica found no evidence of functional brain damage. Damage to white blood cells has also been observed in the laboratory, but again, the practical importance of this is unclear. Whatever temporary changes marihuana may produce in the immune system, they have not been found to increase the danger of infectious disease or cancer. If there were significant damage, we might expect to find a higher rate of these diseases among young people beginning in the 1960s, when marihuana first became popular. There is no evidence of that. A large multicenter AIDS cohort study involving nearly five thousand homosexual men who were followed for eighteen months found no correlation between use of marihuana and immune status. Furthermore, use of cannabis had no effect on the speed of the progression of human immunodeficiency virus disease.[25]

24. Carter and Doughty, "Social and Cultural Aspects"; Rubin and Comitas, *Ganja in Jamaica;* Stefanis, Dornbush, and Fiuk, *Hashish.*

25. R. A. Kaslow, W. C. Blackwelder, D. G. Ostrow, D. Yerg, J. Palenicek, A. H. Coulson, and R. O. Valdiserri, "No Evidence for a Role of Alcohol or Other Psycho-

Another issue is the effect of marihuana on the reproductive system. In men, a single dose of THC lowers sperm count and the level of testosterone and other hormones. Tolerance to this effect apparently develops; in the Costa Rican study, marihuana smokers and controls had the same levels of testosterone. Although the smokers in that study began using marihuana at an average age of fifteen, it had not affected their masculine development. There is no evidence that the changes in sperm count and testosterone produced by marihuana affect sexual performance or fertility.

In animal experiments THC has also been reported to lower levels of female hormones and disturb the menstrual cycle. When monkeys, rats, and mice are exposed during pregnancy to amounts of THC equivalent to a heavy human smoker's dose, stillbirths and decreased birth weight are sometimes reported in their offspring. There have also been reports of low birth weight, prematurity, and even a condition resembling fetal alcohol syndrome in some children of women who smoke marihuana very heavily during pregnancy;[26] other studies fail to demonstrate any effect on the fetus or neonate.[27] The significance of these reports is unclear because controls are lacking and other circumstances make it hard to attribute causes. To be safe, pregnant and nursing women should follow the standard conservative recommendation to avoid all drugs, including cannabis, that are not absolutely necessary for their well-being.

After carefully monitoring the literature for more than two decades, we have concluded that the only well-confirmed deleterious physical

---

active Drugs in Accelerating Immunodeficiency in HIV-1-positive Individuals," *JAMA* 261 (1989): 3424–3429.

26. R. Hingson, J. Alpert, N. Day, E. Dooling, H. Kayne, S. Morelock, E. Oppenheimer, and B. Zuckerman, "Effects of Maternal Drinking and Marijuana Use on Fetal Growth and Development," *Pediatrics* 70 (1982): 539–546; Q. H. Qazi, E. Mariano, E. Beller, D. Milman, W. Crumbleholme, and M. Buendia, "Abnormalities in Offspring Associated with Prenatal Marijuana Exposure," *Pediatric Research* 17 (1983): 1534.

27. P. A. Fried and C. M. O'Connell, "A Comparison of the Effects of Prenatal Exposure to Tobacco, Alcohol, Cannabis and Caffeine on Birth Size and Subsequent Growth," *Neurotoxicology and Teratology* 9 (1987): 79–85; P. A. Fried, "Postnatal Consequences of Maternal Marijuana Use in Humans," *Annals of the New York Academy of Sciences* 562 (1989): 123–132.

effect of marihuana is harm to the pulmonary system. Smoking narrows and inflames air passages and reduces breathing capacity; some hashish smokers seem to have damaged bronchial cells. Marihuana smoke burdens the lungs with three times more tars (insoluble particulates) and five times more carbon monoxide than tobacco smoke. The respiratory system also retains more of the tars, because marihuana smoke is inhaled more deeply and held in the lungs longer.[28] On the other hand, even the heaviest marihuana smokers rarely use as much as an average tobacco smoker. So far, not a single case of lung cancer, emphysema, or other significant pulmonary pathology attributable to cannabis use has been reported in this country.

Furthermore, the risk can be reduced. One way would be to increase the potency of the marihuana used in medicine so that less smoking would be necessary and the lungs would be less exposed to toxins. A higher potency would not necessarily heighten other dangers of marihuana, because, as we have noted, smokers find it easy to titrate the dose, stopping when they attain the desired effect. Another way to reduce the risk is the use of water pipes and other filtering systems, which are now foolishly discouraged by the law. If marihuana were legal, there would be strong incentives to develop further technologies for the separation of undesirable from desirable constituents of cannabis smoke.

Robert Randall, who has now been smoking ten marihuana cigarettes a day for more than fifteen years as a treatment for glaucoma, has this to say about its medical risks and benefits:

> The power of modern propaganda is evident in the question seemingly intelligent people ask about my long-term use of marihuana. An example: after I have spoken with a reporter for three hours, while cogently relating a myriad of compound facts in a high-density, linear, time-sensitive chronology, the reporter

28. T.-C. Wu, D. P. Tashkin, B. Djahed, et al., "Pulmonary Hazards of Smoking Marihuana as Compared with Tobacco," *New England Journal of Medicine* 318 (1988): 347–351; D. P. Tashkin, B. M. Calvarese, M. S. Simmons, et al., "Respiratory Status of Seventy-four Habitual Marijuana Smokers," *Chest* 78 (1980): 699–706.

will suddenly switch subjects: "Has marihuana adversely affected your memory?" How can one reasonably respond to such a question? . . . . It reminds me of the aggressive prosecutor who, after ranting endlessly on the hazards and horrors occasioned by chronic cannabis consumption, abruptly departed from his diatribe to accuse me of being a "very articulable" fellow. Articulation is, of course, the precise antithesis of scrambled synapse, the hallmark of a well-ordered brain at work. So one wonders what the prosecutor was actually asking . . . .

There is a second range of questions dealing with purely physiologic concerns. These questions are often advanced by adolescent males who, as might be expected given the population, favor questions relating to ill-disguised sexual concerns. Despite my chronic long-term high-dose use of marihuana, there is no gross evidence of unusual breast development. I still shave at least once a day, my voice remains comfortably masculine, and despite advancing age, my sperm are as frisky as ever. Occasionally I even display profoundly territorial instincts. . . .

Of all the concerns, respiratory considerations strike me as the most obvious. We are conditioned by decades of propaganda to assume inhaling smoke causes cancer, always. This is not, of course, the case. . . . But let us suppose this leap into the unknown is correct; that constant, long-term, high-dose marihuana use may in some number of people, result in pulmonary or respiratory complications. What does this tell us? People with life- and sense-threatening diseases are routinely confronted by stark choices. On the one hand are the devastating consequences of a debilitating, progressive disease. On the other loom the unwanted, often highly damaging biological and mental consequences of the toxic chemicals required to check the progression of disease. This is called balancing risks and benefits. It is something all seriously ill people contend with every day of their therapy. Viewed in this medical context, marihuana is more benign and far less damaging than the synthetic toxins routinely prescribed by physicians . . . .

Marihuana has helped preserve my vision for more than fifteen years. If, with advancing age, I encounter a serious, as yet unrealized complication, such are the breaks. It is a risk I am willing to take. As W. C. Fields noted, "Life's dangerous. You are lucky to get out of it alive." In the real world, where I live, seeing is the benefit I derive from my chronic association with cannabis. On the negative side there is thankfully little to report. Nothing really. There has been no gross loss of mental capacity. There is nothing physically alarming, distressing, or even mildly annoying. . . . If confronted with a choice between vision and mental agility, agility would win. Smoking marihuana has not confronted me with such a stark choice. Instead, this humble herb has offered me many years of prolonged sight at little cost to my sanity or security.

4 The Once and Future Medicine

There is overwhelming evidence that the American people think medical marihuana should be available to them. In early 1990 a scientifically valid poll conducted by a major survey research firm for the Drug Policy Foundation, an organization working for the reform of drug laws, found that 69 percent of those polled thought doctors should be allowed to prescribe marihuana for glaucoma. In July 1991 the Louisiana legislature voted to recognize the medical value of marihuana in the treatment of paraplegic pain and muscle spasms. By a vote of six to one, in October 1991 the Cambridge, Massachusetts, City Council approved a "home rule petition" that would allow physicians to prescribe marihuana after approval by the state government. A month later 79 percent of San Francisco voters approved an initiative legalizing prescription use of hemp products for any purpose. City officials have said that if state and federal authorities do not intervene, patients who receive prescriptions would be permitted to grow up to six plants on their own. In 1992 Massachusetts became the thirty-fifth state to pass legislation permitting medical use of marihuana.

Reformers have worked mainly within the present regulatory system to get marihuana approved as a legitimate medicine. It would be highly desirable if that could be accomplished, but it seems unlikely. The established federal system for certifying drugs is designed to regulate the commercial distribution of drug company products and to protect the public against false or misleading claims about their efficacy or safety. The term *drug* generally refers to a single synthetic chemical that has been developed and patented, usually by a pharmaceutical company. The sponsor submits an IND application to the Food and Drug Administration and begins testing, first for safety and then for clinical efficacy. When the studies are completed the company asks the FDA to approve a New Drug Application (NDA). To demonstrate effectiveness, the company is supposed to present evidence from controlled studies, not just isolated case reports, expert opinion, or clinical experience. The standards have been tightened since the present system was established in 1962. Although legal rules are technically the same, few NDAs that were approved in the early 1960s would be approved today on the basis of the same evidence. The average time for approval of an NDA is now three years.

The research is expensive, and its cost is borne by the pharmaceutical company, which may spend two hundred million dollars or more before a chemical appears on pharmacy shelves. The company will invest that large sum only if it is reasonably sure that the chemical will succeed as a medicine and the medicine will earn a profit. It has seventeen years to recover its investment.[1] Marihuana will probably never be approved by this process. One reason is that it cannot be patented. Another is that it is a plant material containing many chemicals rather than a single chemical (as we have noted, synthetic THC is available as a prescription drug, but most patients regard it as less effective than whole cannabis). A third reason is that marihuana is taken chiefly by smoking. No drug in the present pharmacopoeia is delivered by this route.

It is an ironic situation. More is known about the adverse effects and therapeutic uses of marihuana than about most prescription drugs. Cannabis has been tested by millions of users for thousands of years and studied in hundreds of experiments sponsored by our own gov-

---

1. In the United States, pharmaceutical products are protected by patent for seventeen years.

ernment over the past thirty years. It is one of humanity's oldest medicines, with a remarkable record of both safety and efficacy. Yet the FDA is legally required to classify it as a "new drug" and demand the same testing it would require for an unknown substance.

Even if whole cannabis somehow became available as a prescription drug, the DEA would classify it in the same way it now classifies THC, as a Schedule II substance with a high potential for abuse and limited medical use—the most highly restricted class of prescription drugs. Restrictions on Schedule II drugs (and all controlled substances) are becoming tighter. Nine states now require doctors to make out prescriptions for many of these substances in triplicate so that one copy can be sent to a centralized computer system that tracks every transaction involving these drugs.[2] Similar legislation is pending in other states.

In 1989 New York State added a group of Schedule IV drugs, the benzodiazepines, to the list of substances monitored in this way. The resulting surveillance of physicians has already had an effect. Research shows that many New York patients with a legitimate need for benzodiazepines are being denied them. Several reports note a rise in the prescription of substitutes that are not as safe or effective. A minimal decline in benzodiazepine overdoses has been more than balanced by an increase in meprobramate, chloral hydrate, ethclorvynol, and glutethimide overdoses. Only 6.7 percent of benzodiazepine overdoses but 22 percent of non-benzodiazepine overdoses were considered to be of moderate or major severity.[3]

2. "State Multiple Prescription Programs," *State Health Legislation Report of the American Medical Association* 16 (August 1988): 35–39.

3. H. I. Schwartz, "Negative Clinical Consequences of Triplicate Prescription Regulation of Benzodiazepines," *New York State Journal of Medicine* 91 (November 1991):9S–12S; H. I. Schwartz, "An Empirical Review of the Impact of Triplicate Prescription of Benzodiazepines," *Hospital and Community Psychiatry* 43 (April 1992): 382–385; M. Weintraub, S. Singh, L. Byrne, et al., "Consequences of the 1989 New York State Triplicate Benzodiazepine Prescription Regulations," *JAMA* 266 (1991): 2392–2397; R. S. Hoffman, M. G. Wipfler, M. A. Maddaloni, et al., "Has the New York State Triplicate Benzodiazepine Prescription Regulation Influenced Sedative-Hypnotic Overdoses?" *New York State Journal of Medicine* 91 (1991): 436–439.

In such a situation physicians can be afraid to recommend what they know or suspect to be the best treatment because they might lose their reputations, careers, and licenses. Even if marihuana were available as a Schedule II drug, pharmacies would be reluctant to carry it and physicians to prescribe it. Through computer-based monitoring, the DEA could know who was receiving prescription marihuana and how much. It could hound physicians who, by its standards, prescribed cannabis too freely or for reasons it considered unacceptable. The potential for harassment would be extremely discouraging. Unlike other Schedule II drugs, such as cocaine and morphine, cannabis has many potential medical uses rather than just a few. Many people would undoubtedly try to persuade their doctors that they had a legitimate claim to a prescription. Doctors would not want the responsibility of making such decisions if they were constantly under threat of discipline by the state. Furthermore, many physicians would not consider prescribing cannabis at all, because they are victims of the government's misinformation campaign. Some still believe and promote such hoary myths as the notion that marihuana is addictive or leads to the use of more dangerous drugs.

Another problem is diversion. The cost of producing cannabis is about a dollar an ounce, and medical distribution would add at most a few dollars more. There are about sixty marihuana cigarettes in an ounce, and the average dose is one cigarette or less. Since the government could not tax a drug used for medical purposes, medical marihuana would cost only a few cents a day. But marihuana on the street is worth its weight in gold—about two hundred to six hundred dollars an ounce. The gap would create a powerful incentive for diversion.

For all these reasons, making marihuana available as a Schedule II drug is likely to be unworkable. That leaves the only program now providing medical marihuana, the Compassionate IND. Since its inception, only about forty of the thousands of patients who might benefit from medical cannabis have been approved for a Compassionate IND; only nine are actually receiving cannabis, and their supplies are often interrupted or of poor quality. The government has now decided not to provide cannabis to anyone else in the future—not even to the patients whose INDs have already been approved. That action is cruel to the few people who might have received government cannabis, but in a broader perspective its effect is marginal and largely symbolic. The government could never have met every legitimate claim through this program without hiring a huge administrative staff, finding an army of physicians prepared to take on the heavy paperwork burden, and convincing patients that they should tolerate endless delays instead of finding marihuana on the street.

In theory, all the therapeutic properties of cannabis could be used if individual cannabinoids in addition to THC were isolated and made available separately as medicines. But this would be an enormously complicated procedure. Sponsors would have to determine the therapeutic potential and evaluate the safety of sixty or more substances, synthesize each one found to be useful, and package it as a pill or aerosol. Since some of these substances probably act synergistically, it would also be necessary to look at various combinations of them. We have already explained why no drug company would provide the resources needed for such a project.[4]

The most recent opening for medical marihuana was a bill introduced in the Maine state legislature in the spring of 1992. Although modeled in part on the state programs of the 1970s and 1980s, this law went further. First, it allowed citizens to defend themselves under state law against criminal charges of marihuana cultivation or possession by showing that they had a diagnosis of glaucoma or were suffering from serious nausea or vomiting from cancer treatment. Sec-

---

4. This is not to say that individual cannabinoids besides THC might not be developed for some medical purposes. We have mentioned that cannabidiol may be an effective antianxiety drug, soporific, antiepileptic, or antidystonic. Resources might be found to develop it through the federal government's orphan drug program or through a use patent (one that protects a new application of a known pharmaceutical product for seventeen years).

Further, the discovery of cannabinoid receptor molecules in the brain suggests that the body itself produces related substances. Compounds might be developed (or discovered) that respond to various subtypes of the cannabis receptor, separating out the therapeutic and other effects of cannabis constituents.

ond, the "therapeutic research program" established by the state was required only to "consider" federal laws. Specifically, if NIDA refused to supply marihuana, the state would use marihuana confiscated by local police. Physicians approved by a special review board would prescribe it to patients who were (1) being treated for glaucoma or undergoing chemotherapy for cancer, (2) in danger of going blind or dying, and (3) not responding to conventional treatment or suffering severe side effects from conventional treatment. Unfortunately, after some favorable votes, the bill was eventually defeated.

We favor any proposal that allows some progress toward medical marihuana use, and we would like to see a program of this kind work, but we are not optimistic. Because the Maine legislation threatened to bypass the federal regulatory system, a conflict would certainly have arisen. The federal government is unlikely to allow its hard-won authority over drug regulation to revert to the states. In any case, the Maine program would have been highly limited; it would have applied to only two of the many potential medical uses of marihuana, and even then only in restricted circumstances. Such programs would be useful if they were extended to include larger numbers of patients with a variety of symptoms. But then the problem of diversion that we have already discussed would arise again, and the federal government would almost certainly intervene vigorously.

Although proposals of the kind embodied in the Maine law do not offer a long-term solution to the problem of medical marihuana, they do have a use. If they are adopted in several states, the federal government will face a political challenge, a needed debate will ensue, and public attention will be drawn to the importance of the issue.

Before we propose a solution to the dilemma of medical marihuana, we wish to examine some of the deeper reasons why so many legal and institutional obstacles have been erected against it. Drug use has been assigned to various social categories, including magic, religion, medicine, self-enhancement, and recreation. Contemporary industrial societies try to keep these categories separate, and the separation is reflected in their formal and informal institutions. Above all, they try to distinguish medical uses of a drug from all other uses.

Like cannabis, most psychoactive drugs now severely restricted by law have had significant medical uses at some places and times. These drugs have tended to fall into disuse as their dangers are more strongly emphasized, other treatments become available, and governments place more controls on the practice of medicine. The history of social and legal responses to the use of these drugs is riddled with examples of hypocrisy, corruption, inadequate pharmacology, inconsistent responses based on inadequate information, indulgence of various social prejudices in response to drug scares, and institutional self-aggrandizement by drug enforcement agencies. But there is a worldwide trend more significant than any of these details. All nations have similar drug laws, which are supplemented by international treaties and drug control agencies.

In the nineteenth-century United States there were almost no government controls on drug use. The growth of manufacturing, capitalist entrepreneurship, and the spirit of liberal individualism made that period an age of self-medication and competing medical authorities. Almost anyone was free to sell almost anything as a medicine. The patent medicine industry flowered, and many of its products contained psychoactive drugs, especially alcohol, opium, and cocaine. Orthodox physicians also used these drugs. Hospital pharmacies stocked large amounts of wine. As late as 1910, morphine was estimated to be the fourth most commonly used medicine, and alcohol was fifth.[5]

Some of the psychoactive drugs, like much strong medicine, could also be powerfully poisonous. Their dangers (as well as their effectiveness) were magnified by isolation of the active chemicals in pure form and the development of such technologies as the hypodermic syringe, which permitted intravenous injection. Mistrust of these drugs had begun to grow by the beginning of the twentieth century. The drugs had been used freely without a careful distinction between health and other purposes—an ambiguity that now began to seem dangerous.

Advances in the art and science of medicine paralleled these devel-

5. M. C. Smith and D. A. Knapp, *Pharmacy, Drugs, and Medical Care* (Baltimore: Williams and Wilkins, 1972), 61.

opments. The rise of synthetic chemistry, experimental physiology, and bacteriology created hope for a scientific medicine based on the recognition of specific disease agents for specific diseases. But psychoactive drugs were not specific cures; they relieved suffering in many situations. Their powers began to seem indeterminate and uncontrollable—more reliable than the power of quack medicines but no less dangerous and mysterious. By the early twentieth century the idea was becoming common that these were subtle poisons with intrinsic powers of deception. Even the best informed person could be possessed by them, becoming dependent or addicted. Taking cocaine to feel alert or opiates to relax could no longer be legitimated as a medical treatment.

The new restraints that began to be imposed at the turn of the century resulted from an impulse to clean up society, impose classifications, and reduce disorder. Just as physical hygiene required government measures to prevent infectious disease and professional hygiene required higher standards for medical and pharmaceutical practice, it seemed that intellectual hygiene required clear and enforceable categories for the use of psychoactive drugs. The process that began with restrictions on patent medicines eventually affected even the power of individual physicians to prescribe psychoactive drugs. Controls were placed on the manufacture and distribution of these substances; certain medical uses were carefully defined, and almost all other uses were outlawed.

In the United States the federal government assumed control of psychoactive drugs through the Pure Food and Drug Act (1906), the Harrison Narcotics Act (1914), and the Volstead Act (1919). Although alcohol was excluded in 1933 under intense public pressure, the system has otherwise persisted, and it has been elaborated in a series of laws leading to the Comprehensive Drug Abuse Prevention and Control Act of 1970 and its successors.

Government control over nonpsychoactive therapeutic drugs grew at a different pace and in a different way, but the trend toward centralization and restriction is similar. The assumption has been that free individual choice in this field is becoming largely illusory and pointless. Federal restrictions began with the Food, Drug, and Cosmetics Act of 1938. That law was amended in 1962 to establish the NDA system, under which the federal government has the power to decide which drugs will be legally available to physicians. The decision had been made that even doctors need protection from misinformed or inappropriate uses of drugs. It was entirely consistent with this view for the DEA to argue in the recent marihuana rescheduling case that even widespread approval by physicians was not enough to justify making marihuana legally available as a medicine.

The greatly increased complexity of the pharmacopoeia explains some of the changes that have occurred since the end of the nineteenth century. Free individual choice seemed more justifiable at a time when the average consumer might be thought to have almost as good a claim as anyone to evaluate the safety and usefulness of the few available medicines. It is plausible to say that in the present situation consumers and even physicians can no longer make that judgment for themselves and that authoritative scientific knowledge supplies the needed basis for decisions.

The system of control over nonpsychoactive drugs is based on this model of consumer protection. It is a powerful justification for government control because it usually applies to areas of social life in which individual autonomy seems least valuable. The principle is that in a complex society far more needs to be known than any single person can learn, and there are some things about which the average person cannot make an informed and rational choice without prior safeguards. Under this system, drugs without accepted medical uses can be seen as resembling defective and therefore dangerous machines or toys. Drugs with medical uses are commodities useful as instruments for certain purposes, but only with safeguards to be supplied by manufacturers and distributors under government direction.

Medical regulations are quite properly the strictest of the consumer protection laws, because the dangers involved can be so great and because the seemingly reliable intellectual authority of science supports any regulatory system. A medical definition of drug control provides a stay against confusion and has therefore become important in public thinking. In a poll conducted in the early 1970s, 30 percent of those asked to choose the best of several definitions of drug abuse chose "use for nonintended purpose, nonmedical use" (27 percent chose "excessive use").[6] We expect the rules against taking risks in medicine to be stricter than the rules against taking risks in the pursuit of pleasure, wealth, or ambition. If an activity as dangerous as professional boxing came under medical control, it would certainly be banned, as the American Medical Association wishes.

But even this control system has been considered inadequate for psychoactive drugs. Prohibition of so-called narcotics began long before prescriptions were legally required for ordinary drugs. The government was telling doctors that using opiates to maintain an addict was not a legitimate medical practice for many years before it started to substitute its judgment for that of physicians about the availability of nonpsychoactive drugs. This regime of highly restrictive controls continues. Something more than consumer protection is involved when the laws criminalize even the consumer and require a vast police bureaucracy for their enforcement. We do not fine or jail the patients of someone who practices medicine without a license or the customers of a manufacturer who disobeys consumer protection laws, yet mere possession of cannabis and other illicit psychoactive drugs is a federal crime. The metaphor of war is rarely invoked in the name of consumer protection but constantly used in the assault on psychoactive drugs. The reason is that laws controlling these drugs are ultimately aimed not at consumer protection but at containing what is believed to be a threat to the social fabric and moral order. If the social fabric and moral order are at stake every time someone casually uses a drug, we need no subtle arguments about whether people need to be protected from themselves.

Yet this distinction is never clearly made, because a certain conception of public health seems to include both purposes. Psychoactive drug use evokes the image of a plague or epidemic possibly more

6. National Commission on Marihuana and Drug Abuse, *Drug Use in America: Problem in Perspective* (Washington, D.C.: U.S. Government Printing Office, 1973), 12.

often and more powerfully than any other social problem. That image suggests a moral crusade that is also a public health campaign. The imagery of disease has tremendous social potency; it eliminates most moral and political doubts. Stopping an epidemic of typhoid presents no moral problems, so why should stopping an epidemic of drug abuse present any? Concerns about individual freedom become irrelevant. Preventing disease has been regarded as a government responsibility for more than a century. National and international systems for the control of psychoactive drugs developed along with international institutions devoted to preventing the spread of infectious disease. Here we act even on remote and indirect possibilities of harm, as when we require vaccinations. The vocabulary in which we talk about psychoactive drug use permits a smooth transition from physical and psychological to moral and finally to social health. Consumer safety and morality, amalgamated through references to health and disease, reinforce one another as justifications for control.

But we are much more likely to disagree about what threatens the moral and social order than about what threatens individual physical (or even psychological) health. Individual values differ, and causes are difficult to distinguish from symptoms in the case of such issues as public tranquility or productivity. As a result, public consensus is weak and the laws may seem arbitrary. Common sense on this issue may be nothing more than shared prejudice. Attitudes toward minorities, work, worldly success and failure, sex, and family life may be the real issues in a controversy about drugs. Drugs are symbols charged with cultural tension. Repressed anxieties may be displaced onto drug users as a form of scapegoating. Marihuana, along with psychedelic drugs, was seen as a catalyst of the antiestablishment movements of the 1960s and 1970s. Even today, millions of people simply do not acknowledge the moral authority of the laws against this drug. Some are ambivalent, some are hypocritical, and some are openly or secretly in resistance. The government insists on viewing marihuana as a threat to society, but the very need to use the rhetoric of war may be a sign that the issue is not settled; obviously, many people doubt whether this battle is worth fighting.

Moral consensus about the evil of cannabis is uncertain and shallow. We pretend that eliminating drug traffic is like eliminating slavery or piracy, or like eradicating smallpox or malaria. No one would suggest that we legalize piracy or give up the effort to eradicate infectious diseases. Yet even conservative authorities like the economist Milton Friedman and the editors of the *Economist* of London have suggested legalizing marihuana and other drugs. The official view is that everything possible has to be done to prevent everyone from ever using any of the controlled substances. But there is also an informal lore of drug use—marihuana use above all—that is far more tolerant. Many of the millions of cannabis users in this country not only disobey the drug laws but feel a principled lack of respect for them. The people who tell their stories in this book do not conceal their bitter resentment of laws that render them criminals. They believe they have been deceived, and they have come to doubt that the "authorities" understand much about either the deleterious or the useful properties of this drug.

The undercurrent of ambivalence and resistance in public attitudes toward the marihuana laws leaves room for the possibility of change, especially since the costs of prohibition are also high and rising. The arrest of more than 300,000 people a year on marihuana charges contributes to the clogging of courts and the overcrowding of prisons. Federal, state, and local governments now spend nearly ten billion dollars a year on drug enforcement and hundreds of millions more to house and feed drug dealers and users in local, state, and federal prisons. A third of federal prisoners are now confined on drug charges, many of them on marihuana charges. Drugs enter the United States at a growing rate despite the war effort, which only inflates prices and keeps the franchises of dealers lucrative. Crime and violence are now produced by the black market in drugs as they were produced by the black market in alcohol in the 1920s.

Besides the measurable billions wasted on prohibition, there are costs more difficult to quantify. One of them is lost credibility of government. Young people who discover that the authorities have been lying about cannabis become cynical about their pronouncements on other drugs and disdainful of their commitment to justice. Another frightful cost of prohibition is the erosion of civil liberties. The use of informers and entrapment, mandatory urine testing, unwarranted searches and seizures, and violations of the Posse Comitatus Act (which outlaws the use of military forces for civilian law enforcement) are becoming more common. It is increasingly clear that our society cannot be both drug-free and free.

It is also clear that the realities of human need are incompatible with the demand for a legally enforceable distinction between medicine and all other uses of cannabis. Marihuana use simply does not conform to the conceptual boundaries established by twentieth-century institutions. It enhances many pleasures and has many potential medical uses, but even these two categories are not the only relevant ones. The kind of therapy often used to ease everyday discomforts does not fit any such scheme. In many cases what lay people do in prescribing marihuana for themselves is not very different from what physicians do when they supply prescriptions for psychoactive or other drugs.

Consider the following case: a ninety-two-year-old woman with severe congestive heart failure, hypothyroidism, cerebral artery insufficiency, and glaucoma (among other maladies) complained of insomnia. Her doctor was reluctant to add one more potent medicine to the eight she was already receiving (in the form of twenty-five pills a day), so he suggested that she drink a glass of wine at bedtime— not a conventional solution, but one that was fairly safe and in this case proved effective. Here the doctor was acting like a nineteenth-century physician in treating alcohol as a therapeutic substance. In the nineteenth century he could have recommended one or two minims of a tincture of cannabis for the same purpose. Today, alas, that is impossible, although marihuana might in some cases be safer and more effective.

Marihuana is also used in a quasi-medicinal way to enhance creativity and productivity. A common problem in the treatment of manic-depressive disorder with lithium carbonate is the complaint of patients that the medication robs them of some of their creativity, vitality, and enjoyment of life—one reason so many of them stop taking it even though they know the potentially disastrous consequences. Mild mood elevation (hypomania) often enhances creative thinking, and experiments show that a better mood often produces more original associations and creative problem-solving. Speed of thought and an easy flow of ideas are associated with elevated mood in bipolar patients.[7] Curiously, these are also common features of cannabis intoxication. In the following account a forty-two-year-old health professional explains how she uses marihuana both to enhance creativity and to make continued use of lithium possible—another situation in which medical and nonmedical uses are impossible to separate.

> In my late twenties, while pursuing an undergraduate degree in the medical sciences, I began to experience the debilitating effects of bipolar affective disorder, commonly known as manic depression. For almost ten years I denied the problem and avoided seeking treatment because of a deep-seated irrational fear: I was unwilling to acknowledge mental illness in myself because my father had been hospitalized for schizophrenia most of his adult life. But eventually my physical and mental health began to deteriorate. I had longer depressions and more severe manic episodes; my social and professional life suffered seriously. At the age of thirty-four I realized that I had to face up to my problem, sought treatment, and recovered with the help of lithium carbonate and psychotherapy. Since then I have faithfully taken lithium and have stayed in remission while continuing to grow personally and professionally.
>
> Marihuana has also played an important part in my recovery and continued remission. I started using it regularly in my middle twenties, at about the time I entered college. In my late twenties I moved away from the college community and no longer had access to marihuana. Within a few weeks I realized how helpful

7. K. R. Jamison, "Mood Disorders and Patterns of Creativity in British Writers and Artists," *Psychiatry* 52 (May 1989): 125–134.

it had been in relieving some symptoms of my (still unacknowledged) mood disorder. During episodes of hypomania I feel unpleasant tension in all my skeletal muscles; marihuana relaxed those muscles more effectively and with fewer side effects than alcohol. Luckily, I was able to gain access to marihuana again and resumed using it, taking two or three puffs two or three times a day.

My psychiatrist asked me to stop using marihuana and gave me a prescription for Xanax (alprazolam) instead. To maintain control, I took as little as I could, just as I had done with marihuana. Xanax worked, but it had undesirable side effects, such as dry mouth and sedation. I continued to use marihuana as well, although I now smoked it only once or twice a week. I stopped using Xanax as soon as the lithium took effect.

After my recovery I returned to school and earned an advanced degree in my medical profession. By now, like many people with bipolar disorder, I was noticing that lithium prevented not only hypomanic mood swings but also the state of consciousness associated with creativity. I feared losing my creativity for both personal and professional reasons. I pursue artistic hobbies for relaxation, and my work also benefits greatly from creative insights—for example, recognition of meaningful patterns in diverse data or new perspectives on obstinate problems. For that reason I continue to use marihuana moderately. I smoke it from a small pipe; usually two or three puffs last me three to four hours. Marihuana allows me to attain the creative state of mind that is so precious to me without having to stop taking lithium and risk a relapse. I also continue to find it useful as a muscle relaxant, especially in treating menstrual cramps.

The following story illustrates in still another context the relation between medical and nonmedical uses:

How do I, a seventy-three-year-old retired-to-the-country woman, happen to be a casual marihuana smoker? Simple. What I read and heard in the sixties (when I was in my forties) persuaded me to try it. I simply could not believe that all those dear intelligent young people (including my son) were doing something stupid and destructive. Of course many were, but not, I think, in smoking marihuana. When a friend and contemporary, a musician, offered to introduce me to reefer madness I accepted. That was—imagine!—a quarter of a century ago.

I have been smoking marihuana in all those twenty-five years, sometimes daily, sometimes occasionally. I smoke it because I enjoy the incredible comprehension of music, the heightened perception of color and form, the diminishment of current problems and pressures, the extension of time. If having an hour and Twinkies with funny friends feels like four hours and gourmet food, do I have to go to jail?

As important as the pleasure, though, is what seems to me to be a palliative quality to marihuana. In an accident twenty years ago I suffered two or three broken ribs. Medical advice was to leave 'em alone, they'll come home. At the time I was employed as editor and operations coordinator of a federally funded, university-based education project. All day long I worked hard, up and down, lugging books and printouts and instructional materials, and all day long I suffered excruciating pain from the broken ribs. I would go home at night, have a couple of tokes on a joint, and, pain-free or at least pain-unaware, I would enjoy a few hours with people, go to bed, and sleep. Yes, for me, if I want it to be, marihuana is Halcion. Funny?

Currently I am troubled by itchy eyes and face. I have seen three doctors and two dermatologists, the second of whom is certain that I suffer from a contact dermatitis. He has embarked on a search for the allergen. So far I have had cortisone cream (in varying strengths) prescribed three times. This may well be a degenerative condition. Whatever it is, when I am seriously uncomfortable and the cortisone seems to be insufficient, a few tokes of the smoke of a mild green plant and the itch is not gone but of no concern to me. For this do I pay a ten-thousand-dollar fine, lose my home, and go to jail?

One more thought on this medicinal application of marihuana: My father, deceased, and my mother, ninety-eight, have both had glaucoma. Considering my gene pool, might I be a likely candidate for the disease? I know nothing about the dosage or source of marihuana used in glaucoma therapy, but it occasionally crosses my mind that my longtime recreational use of marihuana may have been helpful in protecting me from developing glaucoma.

Through all the years that I have engaged in criminal behavior, including growing a few evil plants, I have maintained a successful career in writing and teaching writing. My own published work, in addition to uncountable reports, news releases, proposals, etc., includes a respectably published, enthusiastically reviewed novel and several stories and articles in such publications as *Woman's Day* and *McCall's*. Over these same years I have continued my own writing and taught writing and advertising in a junior college and a major university. I have maintained a home, entertained guests, taken full care of my mother for several years, taken care of children from time to time, gained a reputation as a gourmet cook. (I'm not; I simply follow good recipes precisely.) What I am trying to indicate is that my use of marihuana has never been a drain on my productivity or effectiveness. It has only enhanced my enjoyment of life and, as indicated above, helped me through some medical difficulties.

A musician describes his use of marihuana for creative purposes:

Over the years marihuana has served as a creative stimulant to my work as a performer and my more occasional inspirations as a composer. Almost all my choral pieces and songs have been composed partly or wholly under the influence: melodic and rhythmic ideas just pop into my head during relaxed and happy moments—"points of creative release"—and these seminal ideas are formed into a whole composition over a period of days to years.

Marihuana has also helped me as a performer to gain insights into the meaning of musical masterpieces. Practicing new repertoire while using marihuana is not a good idea, since the keen mental concentration needed to learn notes is somewhat impaired. But once I have learned a piece fluently, marihuana enhances my understanding of what it means as an entirety.

On an average practice day, I work in the morning after drinking a few cups of coffee. In the late afternoon I often have a little workout in the gym, then come back to the piano, smoke some marihuana, and practice enjoyably and productively for one or two hours. I never try to perform in public while stoned, but I often listen to music after smoking marihuana, as do many other musicians I know.

I recently saw a television special on the life of Louis Armstrong in which his lifelong affection for marihuana was pointed out. He found it both an inspiration for his music and a balm against life's trials. It works the same way for me; it's one of my best friends (although I would prefer to take it in another form than smoking).

A scientist reports on the contribution of cannabis to his work:

As a scientist I have spent years training the analytical side of my mind. I have learned to be suspicious of my data, to look for ways to test the reasonableness of my results and arrive at the same conclusions by alternative means. It is an active process of mental discipline: idealizing physical situations, making assumptions to formulate a soluble problem, and applying logic to determine the outcome.

What I have sometimes neglected is an awareness of the wider significance of my work and the sense of wonder that led me into the field to begin with. Often I have been unable to see an answer that lies before me. Part of the blame lies in the very training that enables me to do complicated analytical work. To concentrate on the aspects of a problem that I have included in my model, I ignore apparent distractions that sometimes hold the key to a solution. This happens especially when I work with computers, which can do nothing with the mere suggestion or hint that something important has been left out. It is a human habit to go over old ground repeatedly, seeing what you believe to be there rather than what is actually there (the reason people cannot proofread their own writing). I get high for short periods to remedy this problem. It allows me to turn off the rational side of my mind and think creatively (and randomly). It temporarily cancels the limiting effects of my training and allows me to see my work in a different light.

It would be inefficient to follow up these new ideas while high, because I am too easily distracted and my analytical capacity is impaired. Instead, I enjoy the relaxation and keep notebooks recording my thoughts in lists and outlines. Both the relaxation and the observation of otherwise overlooked details have been valuable contributions to my work.

Another scientist who has found cannabis useful tells his story:

I am a forty-year-old geologist who studies the surfaces of planets and moons at a National Aeronautics and Space Administration research center. I began smoking marihuana in high school, partly out of curiosity and partly in response to peer pressure, after observing no ill effects on my friends who used it regularly. Since then I have used it for self-exploration, for religious experiences, and, of course, for pleasure, including enhanced appreciation of sex, music, art, and conversation. But cannabis has done more than that for me; it has actually helped me to acquire a professionally useful skill.

To analyze the underlying structures and history of geological change on a planet or moon, planetary geologists rely on images of landforms and surface markings radioed back from spacecraft. Landforms cannot be understood unless they are perceived in three dimensions by means of stereo images—paired photographs taken from slightly different angles to mimic depth perception.

Most people use mechanical devices—stereo-opticons of one sort or another—to judge depth from stereo photos. The machinery needed to view stereo images of planetary surfaces is particularly awkward and time-consuming to use. A few fortunate people can see three dimensions in stereo photographs without mechanical aids—a skill every planetary geologist would like to have.

When I was an undergraduate, a friend tried for months without success to teach me this skill, and I became convinced that people who said they possessed it were deluding themselves. But one evening we smoked some especially potent marihuana, purely for pleasure. I amused myself by looking at a pair of stereo photographs that had been left in the room. Suddenly the two pictures merged into a single three-dimensional view. It was like a gift from God. Overjoyed, I looked at other stereo pairs and discovered that I could perceive depth in them as well. I spent the rest of the evening gazing at stereo pairs. The next day, when the immediate marihuana effects had passed, I found that I retained the ability. The skill has saved me a great deal of time in consulting and analyzing stereo photos of geological field sites.

I believe my experience illustrates how marihuana can overcome deep conditioning, initiated immediately after birth, that locks us into perceiving reality in very narrow and formulaistically defined ways. Marihuana shares with its stronger psychedelic brethren the power to cleanse the doors of perception and make the world seem as new. Its help in catalyzing the acquisition of a skill useful in my work is only one of the many blessings and insights it has provided.

The criminalization of marihuana use in general and the policies that make marihuana legally unavailable as a medicine are two problems with the same cause and the same solution. Marihuana is caught in a dual web of regulations—those that control prescription drugs in general and the special criminal laws that control psychoactive substances. These mutually reinforcing laws establish a set of social categories that strangle its medical potential. The only way out is to cut the knot by giving cannabis the same status as alcohol—legalizing it for all uses and removing it entirely from the medical and criminal control systems.

Opponents of medical marihuana sometimes say that its advocates are insincere and are only using medicine as a wedge to open the way for recreational use. Anyone who has studied the history of desperate efforts to obtain legal marihuana for suffering people knows that this is false. The attitude falsely ascribed to advocates of medical marihuana is actually a mirror image of the government's attitude. The government is unwilling to admit that marihuana can be a safe and effective medicine because of a stubborn commitment to wild exaggeration of its dangers when used for other purposes. Far from believing that medical availability of marihuana would open the way to other uses, we take the view that free availability of cannabis may be the only way to make its judicious medical use possible. Marihuana should be available for use in much the same way alcohol is now available. As we noted earlier, cannabis conclusively lost its medical status as an almost incidental effect of the Marihuana Tax Act of 1937, which was designed to prevent "recreational" use. The full potential of this remarkable substance, including its full medical potential, will be realized only when we end that regime of prohibition established two generations ago.

Index

Abdominal mesothelioma, 36
ACTH (adrenocorticotropic hormone),
  68, 69–71, 74, 77
Adapin, 123
Addiction (drug): marihuana as treat-
  ment for, 6, 12
Addiction (to marihuana), 8, 146, 147;
  dependence, 74, 106, 146, 147; mis-
  information, 9, 90, 158; tolerance, 6,
  11, 146
Adrenocorticotropic hormone. See
  ACTH
Adriamycin, 24, 37
Africa, 3, 142
AIDS, 13, 21–22, 85–92, 150
AIDS-related complex (ARC), 88–89
Alcohol, 140, 175; addiction, 11, 147;
  toxicity, 138; use of, 75, 161
Alkeran, 24
Allentuck, Samuel, 111, 143
Alliance for Cannabis Therapeutics,
  15, 21
Alprazolam, 102, 169
American Journal of Psychiatry, 11
American Medical Association, 9, 12–13
American Psychologist, x
American Society of Clinical On-
  cology, 39
Amitryptiline, 102, 116
Amotivational syndrome, 149–50

Amsterdam, 89–90
Anecdotal evidence: defense of, 133–36
Anslinger, Harry, 8, 12
Anti-drug campaign, xi, 165
Antihistamines, 109
Antimicrobial effects, 131
Antitumoral effects, 132
Anxiety: side-effect, 20, 39, 40, 141, 142
Appetite stimulation, 6, 12, 21–22, 30,
  86, 92, 123; ACTH and, 70, 71, 77
ARC (AIDS-related complex), 88–89
Armstrong, Louis, 172
Arrests, 18, 22, 49, 56, 65, 66, 87, 100,
  113; annual number of, x, 166; jail
  sentences, 66, 67
Arthur D. Little Company, 13
Asia, 3
Aspirin, 7; heart attacks and, 134;
  side-effects, 8, 108
Asthma, 6, 127–28
Atopic dermatitis, 109–10, 111, 122
Atropine, 88
Azathioprine, 74
AZT (Zidovudine), 21, 85, 86, 87, 88, 89

Baclofen, 68, 78, 82, 83, 84
Barbiturates, 7, 8, 119, 138
Benabud, A., 142
Benzodiazepines, 68, 139, 147, 157
Beta-agonists, 127

Beta-blockers, 40, 107
Bhang variety, 2, 143, 144
Bipolar affective disorder, 168–69
Birch, E. A., 6
Bladder control, 85
BNDD (Bureau of Narcotics and Dangerous Drugs), 13, 14
Bouquet, R. J., 12
Bowman, Karl M., 11, 143
Brain: stimulation, 2–3; surgery, 101
Bromberg, Walter, 143
Bureau of Narcotics and Dangerous Drugs (BNDD), 13, 14
Burns, 131
Burton, Robert: *The Anatomy of Melancholy,* 3
Buspar, 123
Buspirone, 123

Calcium channel blockers, 107
Cambridge (Massachusetts), 155
Cancer: antitumoral effects, 132; pain, 93
Cancer chemotherapy: nausea, 25–30, 33–35, 37, 88, 91, 141, 145, 159; safety factor in, 31, 138, 139; states allowing marihuana for, 18, 160
Cannabidiolic acid, 141
Cannabidiols, 2, 39, 132, 133
Cannabinoids, 2, 15, 159
Cannabinols, 2
Cannabis, 1. *See also* Marihuana
Cannabis Corporation of America, 15
Carbonic anhydrase inhibitors, 41, 46
Caribbean research, 150
Cartilaginous exostosis, 94
Centennial Exposition (*1876*), 4
Chang, Alfred, 38
Charas variety, 2
Chemotherapy. *See* Cancer chemotherapy
China, 3
Chlorambucil, 24
Chlorpromazine, 107
Cisplatin, 24, 28

Clonazepam, 84, 85
Clorazepate, 66
Cluster headache, 106
Cocaine, 147, 158, 161, 162
Codeine, 84, 85, 93, 103, 104, 105, 107, 108
Committee on Cannabis Indica, 5
Compassionate Use IND. *See* IND
Compazine, 25, 29, 33, 130
Compound Q, 87
Comprehensive Drug Abuse Prevention and Control Act (*1970*), 162
Confiscated marihuana: use of, 19, 97, 160
Conjunctival hyperemia, 138
Controlled Substances Act, 13; Schedule I drugs, 13, 14, 16, 17, 21; Schedule II drugs, 13, 14, 15, 157, 158; Schedule III drugs, 16; Schedule IV drugs, 14, 157
Corticosteroids, 68, 74, 109
Cortisone, 110, 170
Costa Rica, 147, 149, 150, 151
Creativity, 123, 167–68, 169, 171–73
Criminalization of marihuana, 174; black market, 20, 48, 98, 158, 166; dilemma of, 19, 20, 31, 47–48, 74, 78, 89, 105, 126, 166; inexperienced users, 40, 53, 54, 141–42; reform, 13, 14, 15, 49, 155. *See also* Arrests
Culpeper, Nicholas, 3
Cyclophosphamide, 24
Cytomegalovirus retinitis, 91
Cytoxan, 24
Czechoslovakia, 131

Dantrium, 68
Dantrolene, 68
Darvocet, 105
Darvon, 108
Davis, J. P., 59
DEA. *See* Drug Enforcement Administration
Demerol, 54, 107
Depression, 6, 12, 115–24, 130, 149

Dermatitis, 170
deRopp, A. S., 12
Desipramine, 116
Desyrel, 79, 123
Dexamethasone, 101, 102, 103, 104
Dexedrine, 119
Dextroamphetamine, 119
Diamox, 46, 54
Diana, Sam, 73
Diazepam, 68, 75, 82, 134, 139, 147
Dilantin, 59, 63, 64, 65, 66, 101,
    103, 104
Dilaudid, 95, 96, 101
Dingell, John, 10
Diphenoxylate, 88
Diphenylhydantoin, 103
District of Columbia, 17
Doxepin, 123
Doxorubicin, 24, 25
Dronabinol, 90, 91. *See also* Marinol
"Dr. Z," 88–91
Drug abuse, 164; campaigns against,
    xi, 165; as symptom, xi, 150. *See also*
    Addiction
Drug companies, 14, 156
Drug control, 162–63. *See also* Con-
    trolled Substances Act
Drug development, 156, 161–63
Drug Enforcement Administration
    (DEA), 14, 15–17, 163; procedures,
    21, 157, 158; regulations, 83
Drug Policy Foundation, 13, 155
Drug testing: mandatory, x; random
    urine tests, x, 112–13, 167
Duborg, Greg, 129–31
Dysmenorrhea, 6
Dystonias, 132–33

EAE (experimental autoimmune en-
    cephalitis), 81
Ear infections, 131
Economist, The, 166
Ecotrin, 107
Edinburgh New Dispensary, The, 3
Elavil, 102, 116, 119

Ephedrine, 108
Epilepsy, 6, 58, 59–67
Epinephrine, 40, 41, 46
Ergot, 107
Ethiopian Zion Coptic Church, 15
Europe, 3, 4
Experimental autoimmune encephalitis
    (EAE), 81

Farber, Sidney, 26
FDA. *See* Food and Drug Administration
Federal Bureau of Narcotics, 8, 12, 13
Florida, 21–22, 57, 100
Food and Drug Administration (FDA),
    16, 18–19; procedures, 17, 21, 99,
    156, 157. *See also* IND
Food, Drug, and Cosmetics Act
    (*1938*), 163
Foscarnet, 91
Foscavir, 91
Frei, Emil, 26, 28
Friedman, Milton, 166

Galen, 3
Ganja variety, 2, 146
Glaucoma, 40–57, 155; intraocular
    pressure, 41–42, 46–47, 49–50, 51,
    52, 54; marihuana as preventative,
    171; side-effects, 145, 146, 152; states
    allowing use of marihuana for, 18, 30,
    159–60
Gould, Stephen Jay, 36–38, 141
Greece: research in, 149, 150
Grinspoon, Danny, 26–28

Halcion, 139
Handwriting sample (from MS patient),
    76
Hanson, Gordon, 63–67
Hare, H. A., 5
Harrison Narcotics Act, 10, 162
Hashish, 2
Hemp, 1, 3, 4, 5, 6, 7
Hepatitis B, 86, 87
Herpes, 132

"High" (altered state of consciousness), 75, 102, 104, 141
HIV (human immunodeficiency virus), 85, 86, 90, 91
Hodgkin's disease, 33
Hydromorphone, 95
Hyperemesis gravidarum, 129
Hypodermic syringe invention, 7
Hypomania, 168, 169

Ifex, 24
Ifosfamide, 24
Illegal status (of marihuana). See Criminalization
Imipramine, 116, 134
IND (Investigational New Drug), 17, 18; approvals, 19, 21, 22–23, 158–59; Compassionate Use, 20, 21, 22, 23, 57, 74, 81, 158; Individual Treatment, 20; obtaining an, 21, 83, 99, 156, 158–59
India, 3, 4, 148; side-effects in, 142, 143; varieties, 2
Indian Hemp Drugs Commission, 148
Insomnia, 6, 79, 128–29, 167
Institute of Medicine, 148
International Chiefs of Police, 15
Investigational New Drug. See IND
Isocarboxazid, 116

Jaffe, Norman, 28
Jamaica: research, 146, 147, 149, 150
Jenks, Kenneth and Barbra, 21–22
John Hopkins University: Wilmer Eye Institute, 50–51
Journal of the American Medical Association (JAMA), 11–12
Jules Stein Eye Institute (UCLA), 50

Kaolin, 88
Kidney failure: nausea and, 130–31
Kleber, Herbert D., 22

Labor pains, 113–14
LaGuardia Commission, 11, 12, 143, 148

Lasagna, Louis, 133
Law: on medical use, 17, 155, 160; reform, 13, 14, 15, 49, 155. See also Criminalization; Legalization; Medical necessity defense; Medical use
Lawn, John, 17
Legalization (of marihuana), ix, 17, 21, 42, 175; approvals, 38, 52, 57; costs under, 158; states with, 17, 18, 33, 155, 160. See also IND; Law; THC
Leukemia, 26–27, 32
Leukeran, 24
Levonatradol, 2
Librium, 110, 121
Lioresal, 68, 78
Lithium, 116, 119, 122, 125–26, 167–68, 169
Longcope, James C., 129
Longitudinal studies, xi
Loperamide, 88
Louisiana, 18, 155

Maine, 159–60
Manic-depressive disorder, 124–26, 167–68
Marihuana, xii; botanical classification, 1, 2; chemical compounds, 2; geographic distribution, 1, 2, 3; potency, 2, 21, 142, 152; production, 158. See also Criminalization; Legalization; Medical use; Side-effect issues
Marihuana Reconsidered (Grinspoon), ix
Marihuana Tax Act (1937), 8–11, 175
Marinol, 38–39, 50, 88, 90–91, 130–31
Marplan, 116
Mason, James O., 22
Mason, Ron, 86–88
Massachusetts, 17, 155
Mattison, J. B., 6, 7
MDMA (3,4-methylenedioxymethamphetamine), 16
Medical necessity defense, 49, 73; first successful, 52; Florida, 22, 57, 100; Maine, 159–60
Medical use, 15–16; criteria, 16; decline

in, 7–8; government suspension of, 159; history of, 2, 3, 4–7; procedures for, 17–20, 21, 56, 99, 156; public opinion, xii, 155, 166
Melorheostosis, 105
Melphalan, 24
Menstrual cramps, 109, 113, 169
Meperidine, 107
Meprobamate, 121
Methaqualone, 95
Methylphenidate, 119
Methysergide, 107
Mexico: varieties, 2
Michigan, 30, 31–33; Marihuana as Medicine Bill, 33
Middle East, 2, 3
Migraine, 1, 6, 7, 106–09, 130, 131
Military use: research on, 13
Miller, Carol, 107–09
Miltown, 121
Minnesota, 65, 67
Minoxidil, 134
Miotics, 41, 45
M'Meens, R. R., 5
Monoamine oxidase (MAO) inhibitors, 116
Mood disorders, 115–16; manic-depressive, 124–26, 167–68. *See also* Depression
Moreau de Tours, Jacques-Joseph, 117
Morphine, 158, 161; substitute, 6
MS. *See* Multiple sclerosis
Mudrane, 108
Multiple congenital cartilaginous exostosis, 94, 98
Multiple sclerosis (MS), 67–81, 84, 128
Music appreciation, 171–72
Musikka, Elvy, 52–57
Mysoline, 63, 64, 65, 66

Nabilone, 2
Narcotics Commission of the League of Nations, 12
Nardil, 116
National Cancer Institute, 18, 38

National Drug Control Policy, 22
National Eye Institute, 49
National Federation of Parents for Drug-Free Youth, 15
National Institute of Drug Abuse (NIDA), 19, 160; procedures, 21
National Organization for the Reform of Marihuana Laws (NORML), 13, 14, 15, 49
Nausea, 88; in AIDS, 21; and chemotherapy, 25–30, 33–35, 37, 88, 91, 141, 159; in kidney failure, 129–31; in pregnancy, 114
NDA (New Drug Application), 156
Negen, Deborah, 32
Neuroleptic drugs, 133
New Drug Application (NDA), 156, 163
New English Dispensatory, The, 3
New Mexico, 17, 18–19
New York, 11, 20; Schedule IV drugs in, 157
NIDA (National Institute of Drug Abuse), 19, 21, 160
Nitrogen mustard derivatives, 24, 25
NORML (National Organization for the Reform of Marihuana Laws), 13, 14, 15, 49
Norpramin, 116, 123
Nortripytline, 130
Nutt, Keith, 28, 29–32, 33

Oglesby, Carl, 60–63
Ondansetron, 25
Opioids, 14, 82, 92, 95, 105, 107, 108
Opium, 161, 162
O'Shaughnessey, W. B., 4, 5
Osler, William, 7

Pain, 4, 5, 7, 170; burns, 131; chronic, 92–106
Palacky University (Czechoslovakia), 131
Paranoia, 40, 141
Paraplegia/quadriplegia, 81–85, 155
Parker, C. S., 117
Parnate, 116

Paufler, Greg, 69–74, 135
Pentazocine, 14
Perception enhancement, 170, 173
Personality changes, 11, 149–50. *See also*
    Psychosis
Peru, 39
Phenelzine, 116
Phenobarbital, 59, 63, 64, 65, 108
Phenothiazines, 143
Phenytoin, 59, 63
Phospholine iodide, 46, 54
Physicians, 104, 163; dilemma, 53, 99,
    158; prescriptions by, 13, 15, 155,
    157; red tape for, 8, 18, 20, 21, 56, 99
Physicians Association for AIDS Care, 13
Physostigmine, 75
Pierson, Lynn, 18, 19
Pilocarpine (Pilo), 41, 45, 46, 53, 54
Platinol, 24
Police: cooperation, 97
Political aspects, 49–50, 165
Pond, D. A., 117
Posse Comitatus Act, 167
Potassium depletion, 71, 72, 102
Prednisone, 68, 71, 107
Pregnancy, 151
Pride Quarterly, xi–xii
Primidone, 63
Prochlorperazine, 25, 88
Promethazine, 88
Propoxyphene, 105, 108
Propranolol, 75, 134
Prostaglandin, 83
Protryptiline, 122
Prozac, 87, 116, 119, 123
Pruritis, 109
Pseudopseudohypoparathyroidism,
    93–94, 98
"Psychiatric Aspects of Marihuana
    Intoxication, The" (Allentuck and
    Bowman), 11
Psychoactive drugs, 2; control of, 161–
    62, 164
Psychoactive effects, 135, 139–45;

preparation for, 40, 93, 142. *See also*
    Side-effect issues
Psychosis, 142–44; drug treatment, 133
Public Health Service, 22
Pupil dilation/constriction, 41
Pure Food and Drug Act, 162

Radiation treatments, 102. *See also*
    Cancer chemotherapy
Ramsey, H. H., 59
Randall, Robert, 21, 42–52, 135, 152–54
Ranitidine, 88, 101
Recreational use, xii, 141; concern about,
    8, 13, 137, 175; tax on, 8
Reefer Madness (film), 8
Religious freedom defense, 15
Reproductive system effects, 151
Research, 41, 149, 156; government, 13,
    156–57; lack of incentives, 156, 159;
    prohibition and, 80, 137
Retin-A, 134
Reynolds, J. R., 6
Ritalin, 119
Rosenfeld, Irvin, 94–101
Ross, Karen, 101–5

Sacred plants, 15
Safety (of marihuana), 31, 74, 136,
    137, 167. *See also* Side-effect issues;
    Toxicity
Safety factor, 138
San Francisco, xii, 155
Schedule I, II, III, IV drugs. *See under*
    Controlled Substances Act
Secobartital, 138
Seconal, 138
Serotonin, 106–7, 109
Sexual function, 11, 74, 75, 83, 84,
    120, 153
Shukla, S. R. P., 143, 144
Side-effect issues, 123, 133, 136–54;
    acute effects, 138–45; anxiety, 20, 39,
    40, 141, 142; chronic effects, 145–54;
    creativity, 123, 167–68, 169, 171–73;

criminality, 8, 9, 11, 164; flashback, 145; hallucinations, 142, 145; "high," 75, 102, 104, 141; mental concentration, 85, 172; mental deterioration, 8, 12, 148, 154; operating machinery, 139–40; personality changes, 11, 149–50; psychoactive, 40, 93, 135, 139–40; pulmonary damage, 152, 153; stepping-stone hypothesis, 147, 158. See also Safety; Toxicity
Single-patient randomized trial, 135
Skin disorders, 109–13, 122, 170
Smoke: marihuana vs. tobacco, 152; passive exposure, x
Smoking (as method), 19, 20, 38–39, 50, 91, 133, 156
Social/political aspects, 49–50, 165
Sopor, 95, 96, 101
South Africa, 3
South America, 3
Southeast Asia, 3
Spear, Don, 109–13, 135
Staphylococcus, 131
Stepping-stone hypothesis, 147, 158
Stereo imaging, 173–74
Steroid therapy, 68–72, 109, 127. See also ACTH; Corticosteroids; Prednisone
Stockings, G. T., 117
Stroup, Keith, 49
Synhexyl, 2

Taft, Harris, 33–36
Talshir, Debbi, 75, 77–78
Talwin, 14
Taxes, 158. See Marihuana Tax Act
Tetrahydrocannabinol, 2, 76, 130–31, 138. See also THC
Thacore, V. R., 143, 144
THC (tetrahydrocannabinol), 2–3, 156; classification of, 14–17; delta-1-, 2; delta-8-, 132; delta-9-, 2, 38, 39, 132; immuno-suppressive effects, 81; legal use, 38; smoked marihuana

vs., 19, 20, 38–39, 50, 91, 133, 156; strengths, 21, 75, 100, 142; synthetic, 2, 18, 38, 39; testing of synthetic, 19, 50, 84–85, 93, 117–18. See also Marinol
Thorazine, 107
3,4-methylenedioxymethamphetamine (MDMA), 16
3,4-trans-delta-1-tetrahydrocannabinol, 2. See also THC
Thyroid hormone, 119
Tic douloureux, 6
Tofranil, 116, 121
Tolerance, 6, 11; behavioral, 146
Toxicity: acute, 137–45; chronic, 137, 145–54; of conventional treatments, 24
Tranxene, 66
Tranylcypromine, 116
Trazodone, 79, 123
Tretinoin, 134
Tricyclics, 116, 118, 119, 122, 123
Tylenol, 103, 104, 105, 108

United Nations Single Convention on Narcotic Substances, 14
United States: marihuana use in, 2, 4
United States Court of Appeals, 14, 16
United States Pharmacopoeia and National Formulary, 8
University of California, xi, 41; Jules Stein Eye Institute, 50–51
University of Göttingen, 75
University of Iowa, 93
University of Miami, 55
University of Minnesota, 65
University of Mississippi, 21
Urine tests, x, 112–13, 167

Valium, 71, 110; side-effects, 65, 66, 68, 72, 83, 139, 147
Victoria, Queen, 4
Vivactil, 122
Volstead Act, 162

Water pipes, 152
Wilmer Eye Institute, 50–51
Winthrop, Roger, 30
Winthrop Pharmaceuticals, 14
Woiderski, Chris, 82–84
Woodward, W. C., 9–11
Wrigley, F. W., 117

Xanax, 102, 103, 139, 169

Young, Francis J., 15–16

Zantac, 101, 122, 130
Zidovudine (AZT), 85–86
Zofran, 25–26, 130